Design Your *Happy*

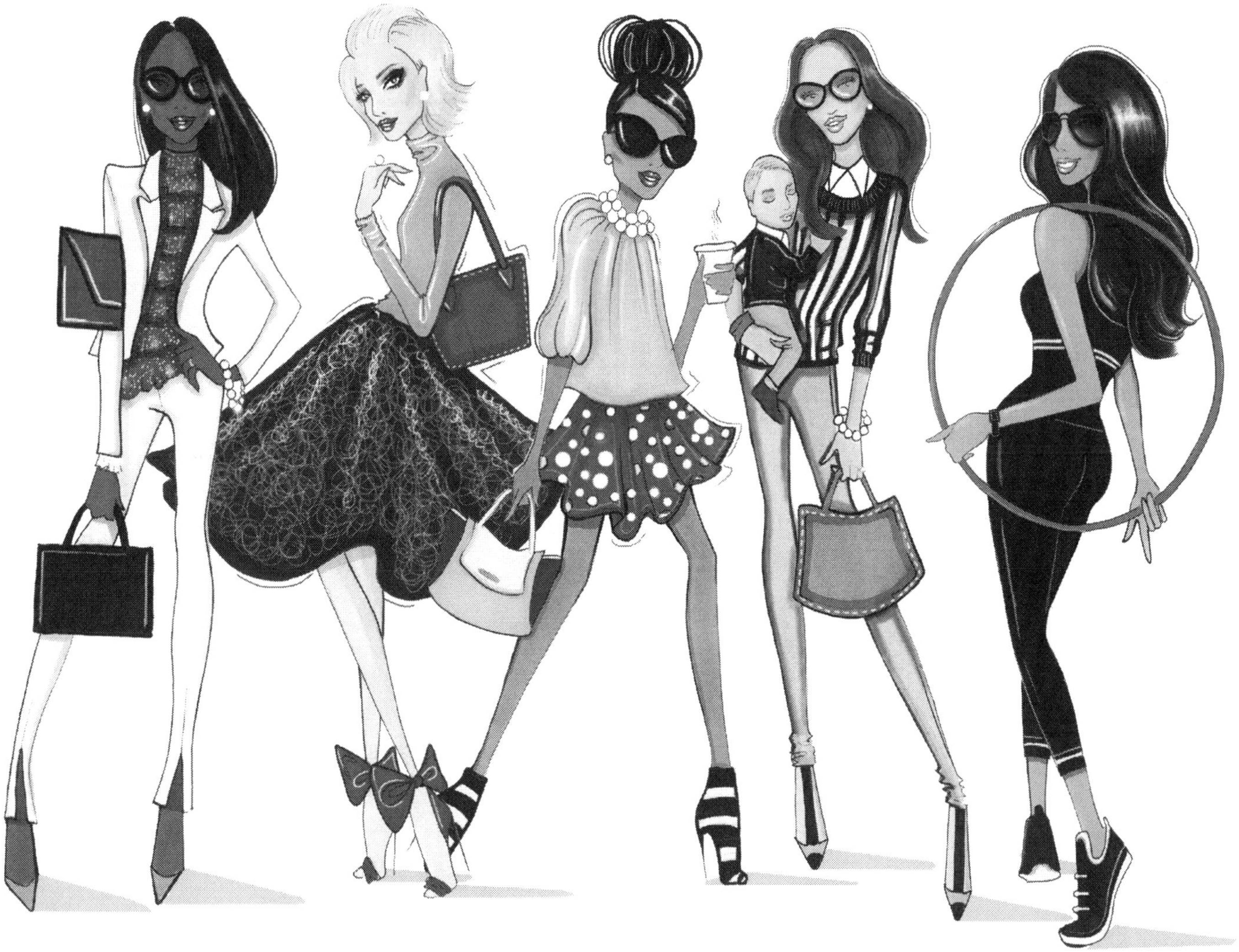

12 WEEKS TO A HAPPIER YOU

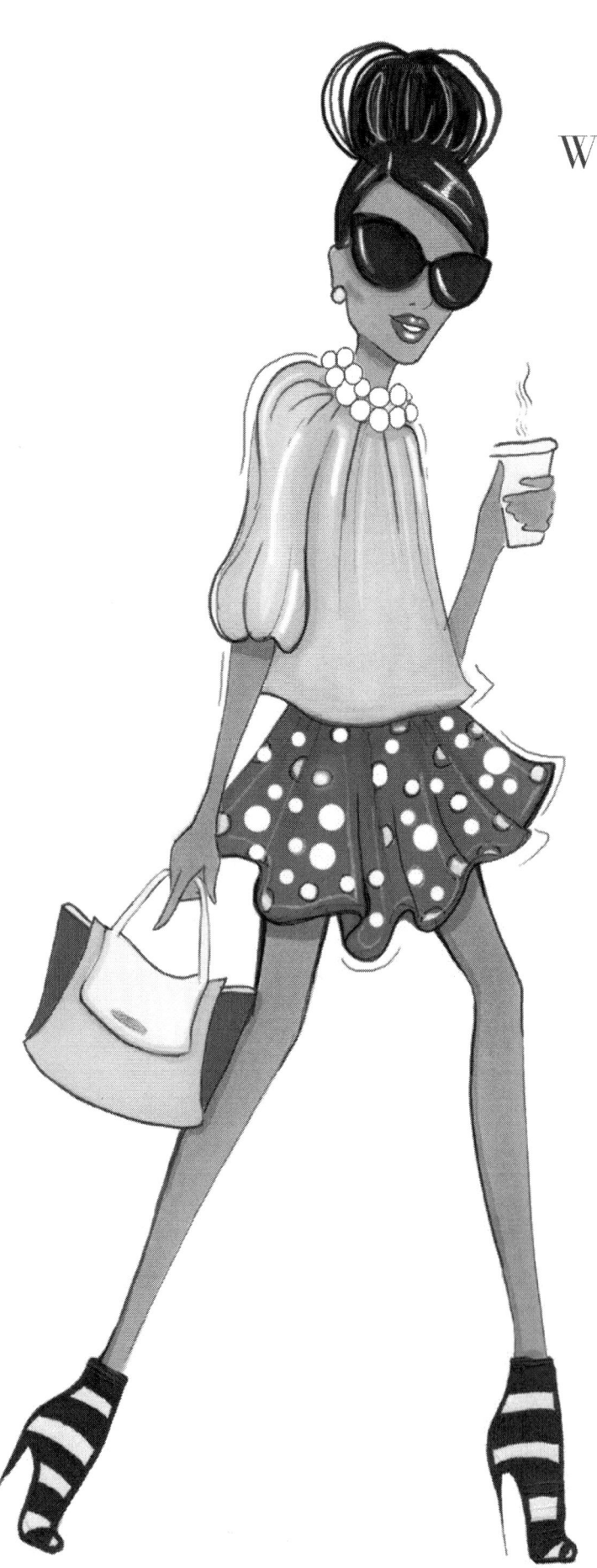

Welcome! Here's how this works...

The theme Scripture for the Design Your Happy Journal is Isaiah 32:8.

"But the noble make noble plans and by noble deeds they stand."

When you work through this journal with God, it will help you find clarity, confidence and success.

It starts out with a Life Design Plan.

Because the only way to get where you want to go is to figure out where that is and map out the path to get there.

So make your noble plan first.

Then every day, invest 5 minutes filling out "your 5" to set your intention, record your wins and stay accountable!

More on that later. But it will help you walk in your noble deeds.

The quote for each day will inspire you to keep going towards building the life you want!

Design your happy. With God.
On purpose.

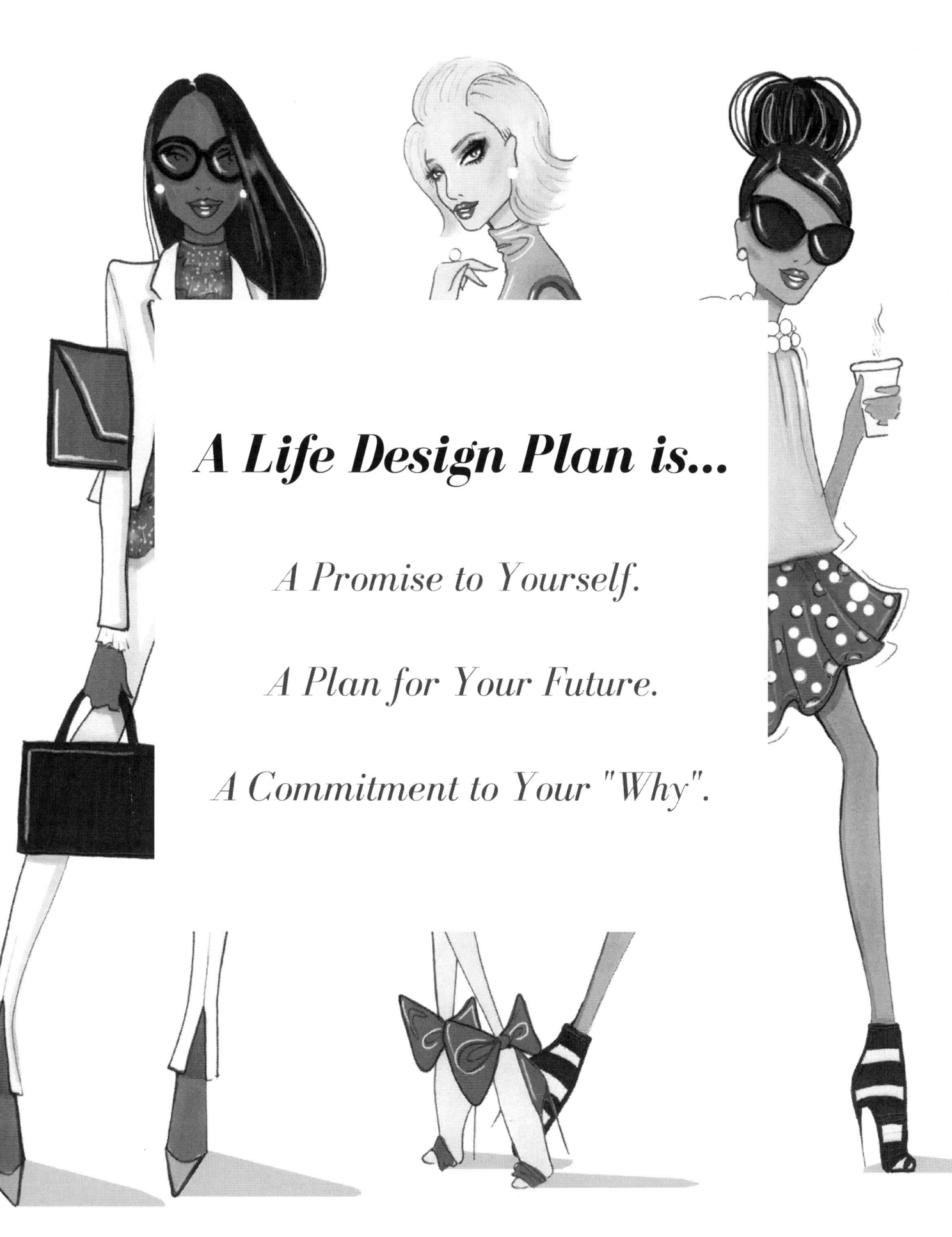

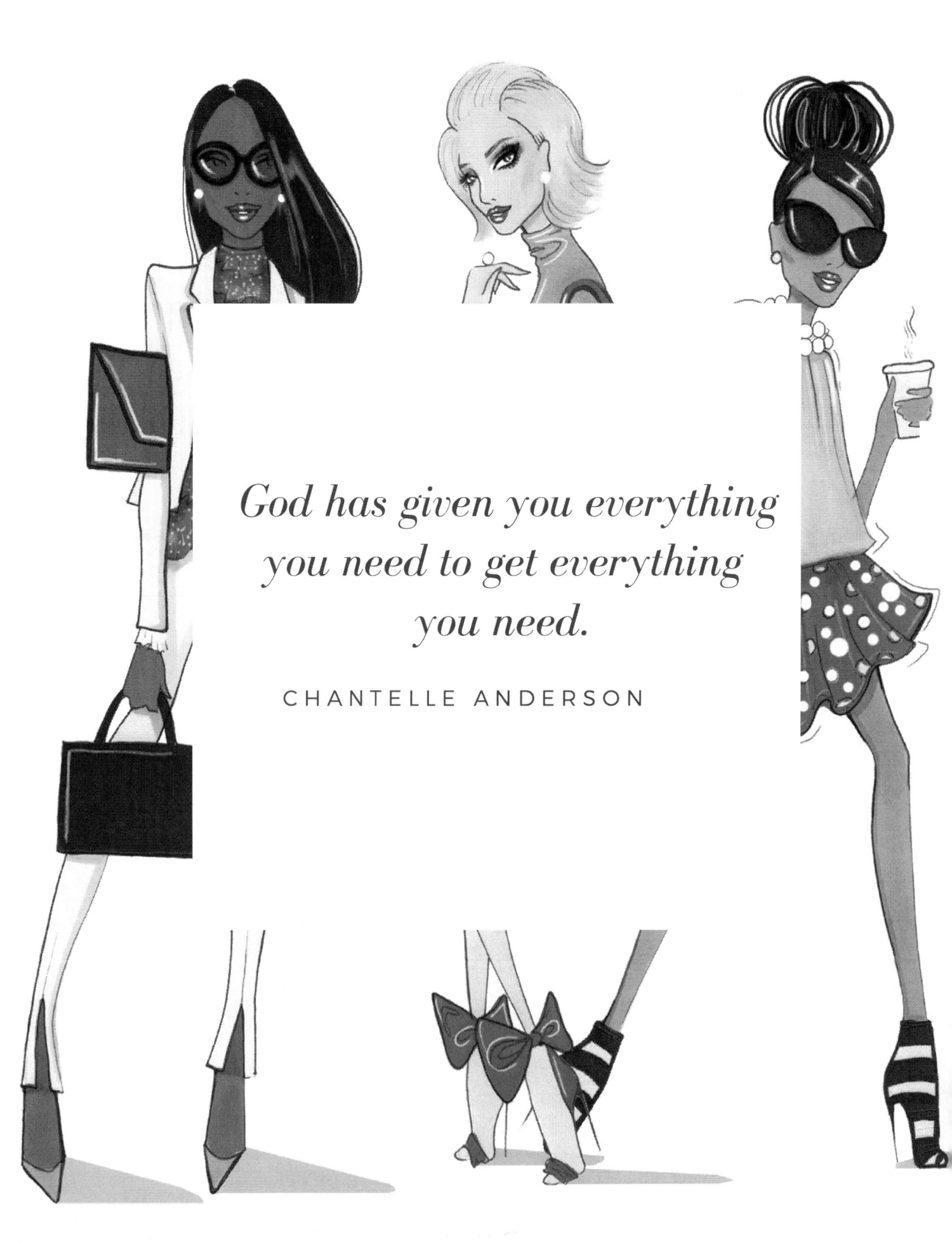

Compartmentalize

THE "ALL" IN YOUR "HAVE IT ALL"

"Take delight in the Lord and He will give you the desires of your heart." - Psalm 37:4
What do you want?
What does your ideal life look like?

_____
_____
_____
_____
_____
_____
_____
_____
_____
_____
_____
_____

Set Your Vibe

THE ROOT NEEDS OF YOUR WANTS

"What a person desires is unfailing love." - Proverbs 19:22

What does the life you want feel like?

_____
_____
_____
_____
_____
_____
_____
_____
_____
_____
_____

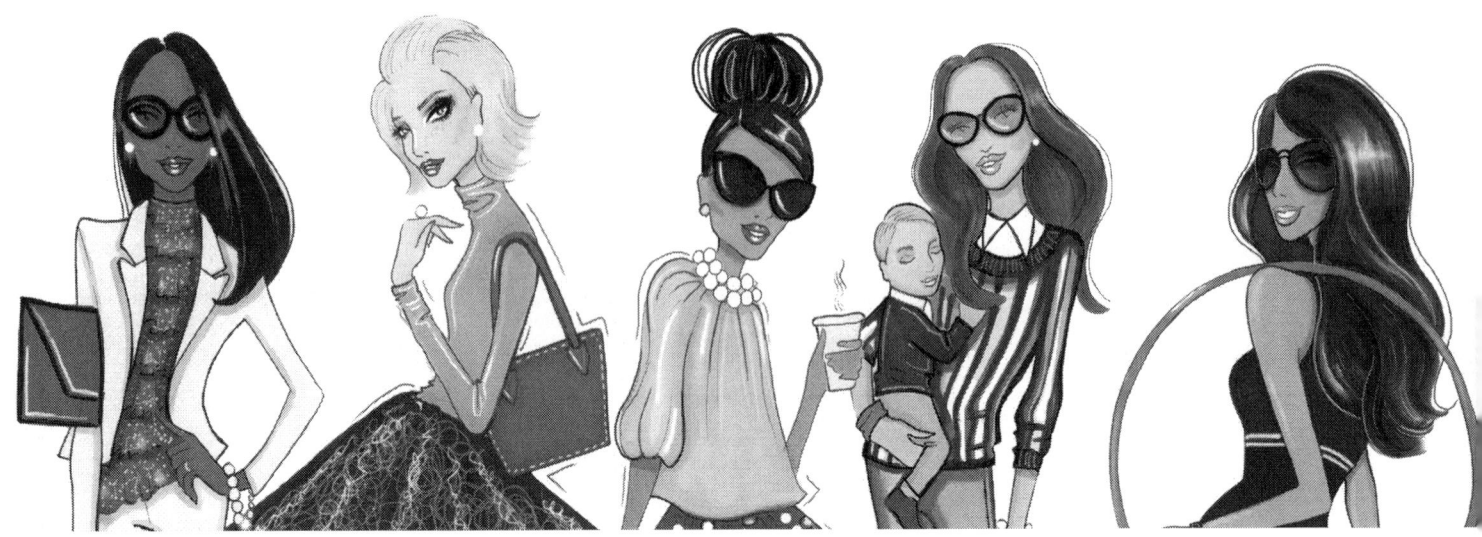

Define Your "Why"

YOUR MOTIVATION FOR SUCCESS

"Whatever you do, do it all for the glory of God." - 1 Corinthians 10:31
When this plan feels impossible, what's going to keep you from quitting?

Find Your Gifts

THE TOOLS YOU HAVE TO BUILD WITH

"We have different gifts, in accordance with the grace given each of us." - Romans 12:6
What comes naturally to you, that you can do for hours that feel like minutes?
What makes your heart ache that your skills can address?

_____
_____
_____
_____
_____
_____
_____
_____
_____
_____
_____

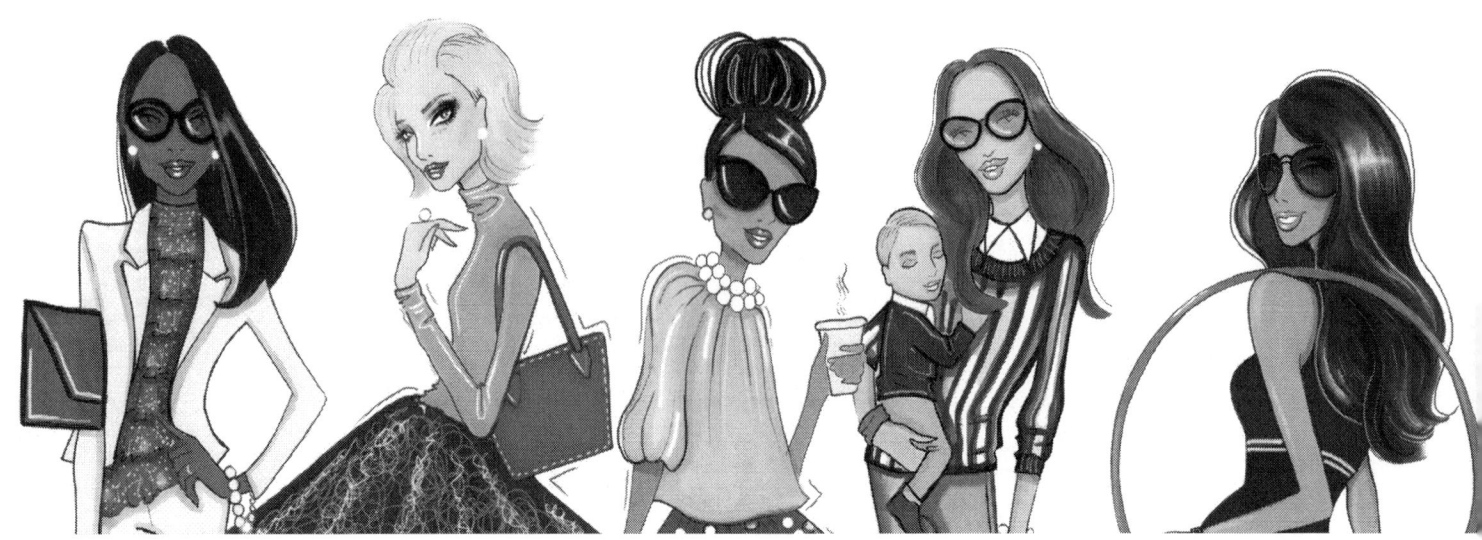

Define Your Brand

WE ALL HAVE A PERSONAL BRAND

"But you are a chosen people, a royal priesthood, a holy nation..." - 1 Peter 2:9
How do you want people to describe you when you're not around?
What is a concise, personal story that people can relate to?

_____
_____
_____
_____
_____
_____
_____
_____
_____
_____
_____

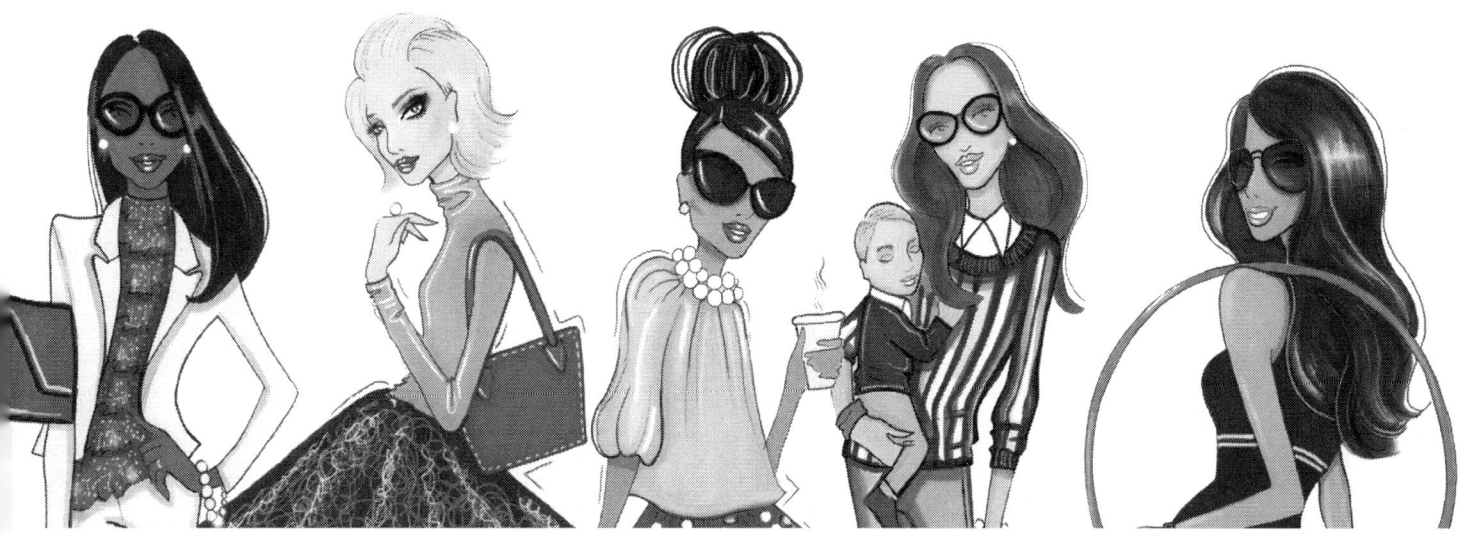

Identify Improvement Areas

PRACTICAL CHANGES NEEDED FOR SUCCESS

"Give careful thought to the paths for your feet..." - Proverbs 4:26
What will I add or take away so I can say "yes" to everything in this plan?
What is going to prevent my success unless I change it?

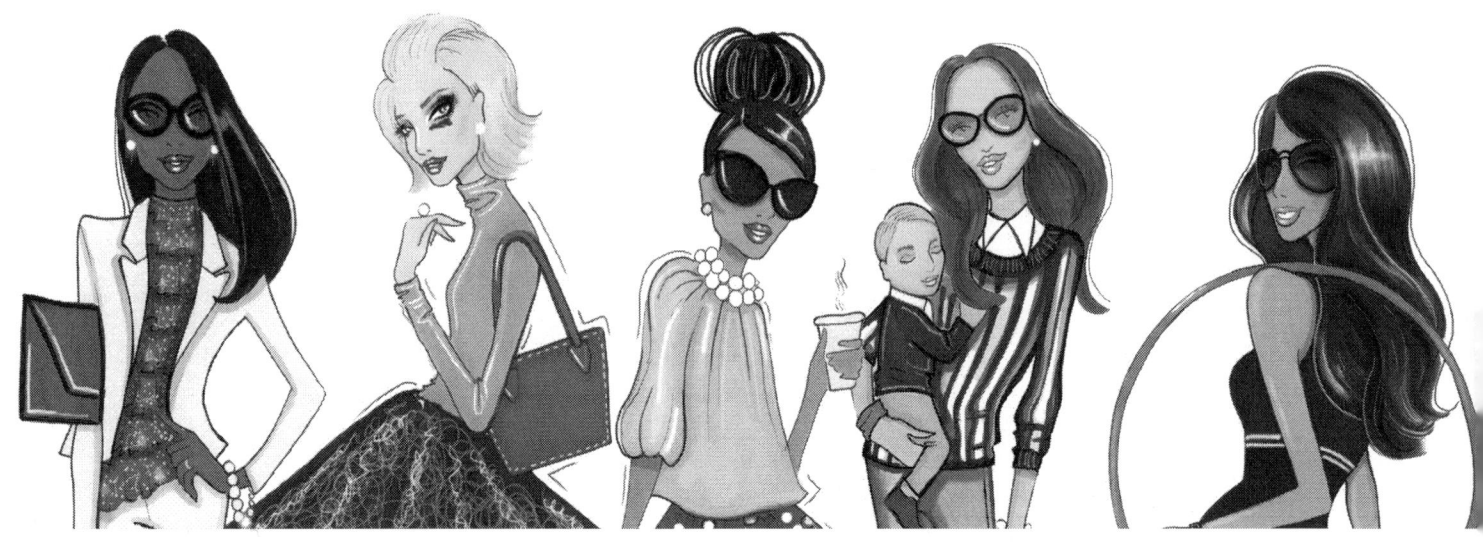

Pick Your Inner-Circle

PEOPLE GOING WITH YOU ON THIS JOURNEY

Do not be deceived: bad company corrupts good character. - 1 Corinthians 15:33

Friends & Family
Love, emotional support, pep talks, first investments. Listen to their input.

-
-
-
-
-
-

Board of Directors
Mentors, coaches, experts in their field, people you imitate. Take their advice.

-
-
-
-
-
-

*How can I continue to build these relationships so that they're all mutually beneficial partnerships?

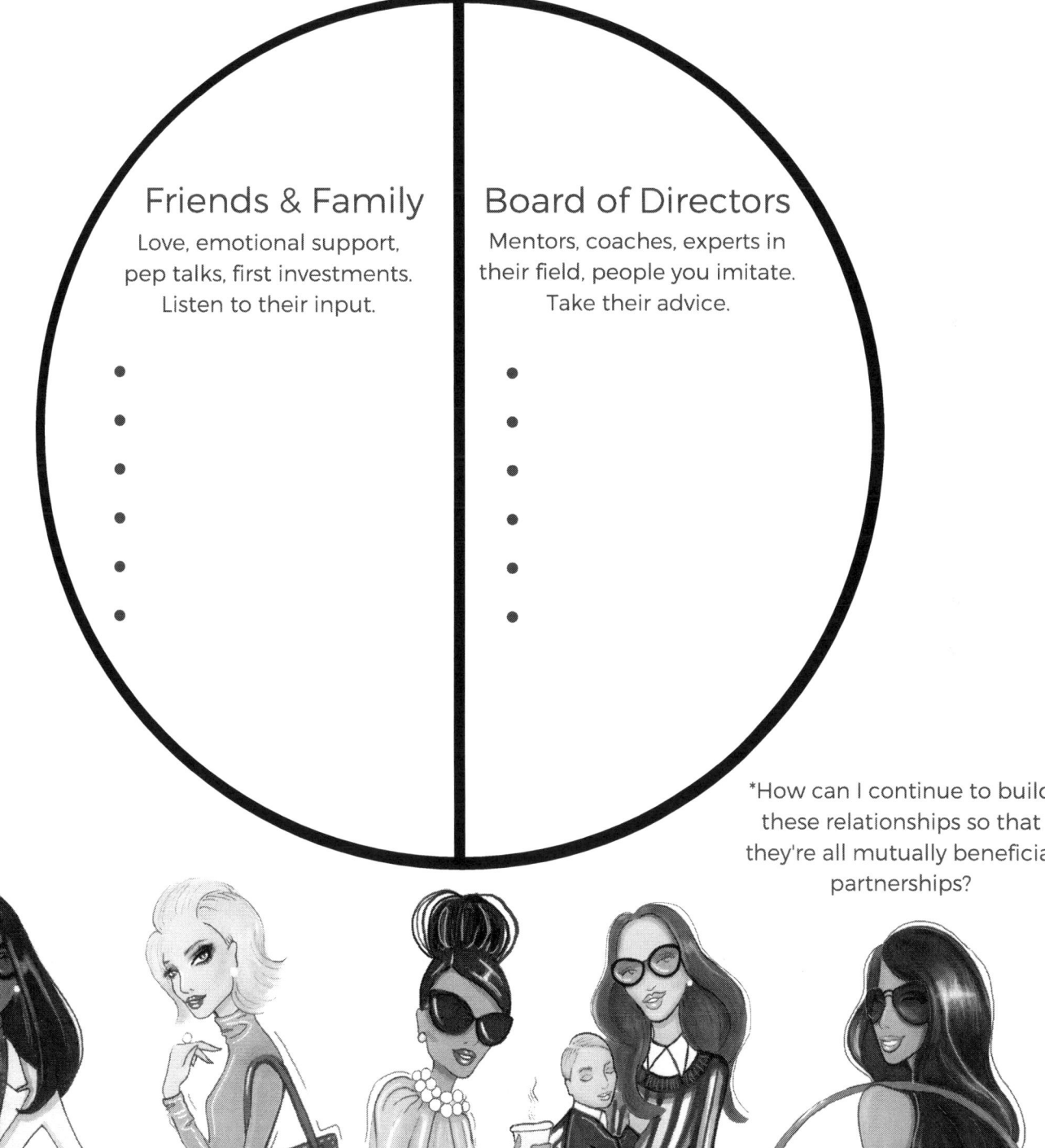

Defend Your Bubble

GUARDING YOUR DREAM

"Can a man scoop fire into his lap without his clothes being burned?" - Proverbs 6:27
What is polluting my space or stealing my energy?
Am I willing to say "no" to sentimentality for the sake of my progress?

_____
_____
_____
_____
_____
_____
_____
_____
_____
_____
_____

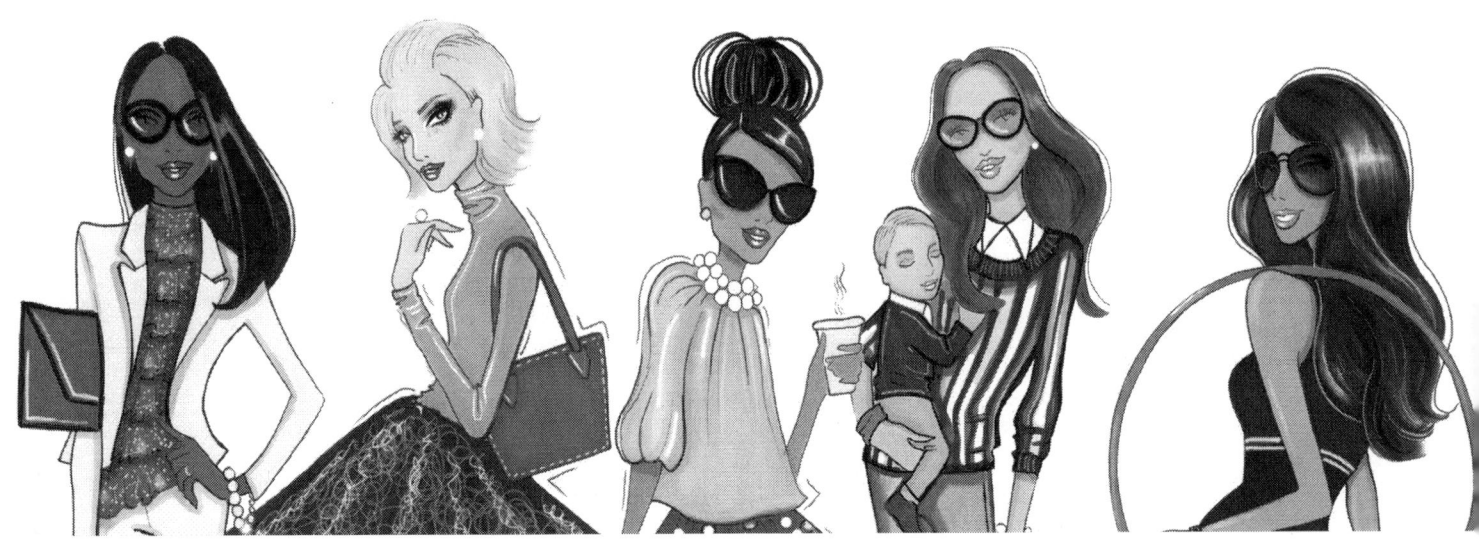

Fill and Refill

PERSONAL AND PROFESSIONAL MAINTENENCE

"Dear friend, I pray that you may enjoy good health..." - 3 John 1:2
What will I do to pamper and take care of myself?
What will I do to continue growing in knowledge, skill and maturity?

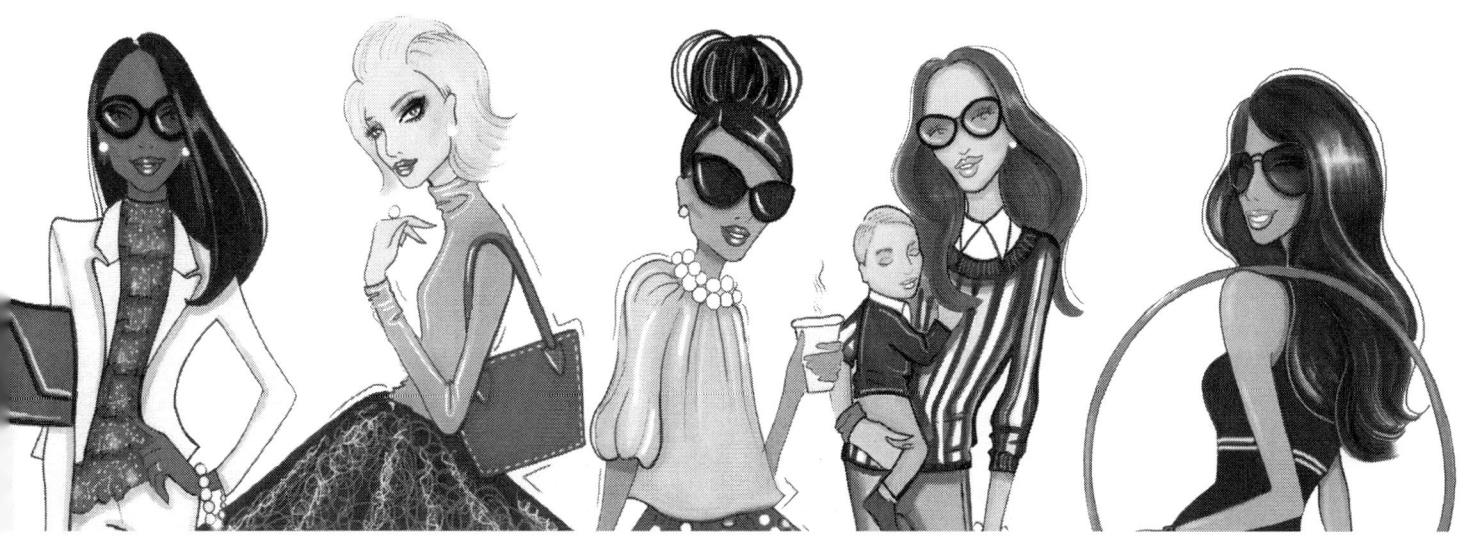

Take Action

IT'S GO TIME!

"For we walk by faith, not by sight." - 2 Corinthians 5:7

What specific steps will I take right now to start creating the life I designed?

What systems will I put in place to make sure I stick to it?

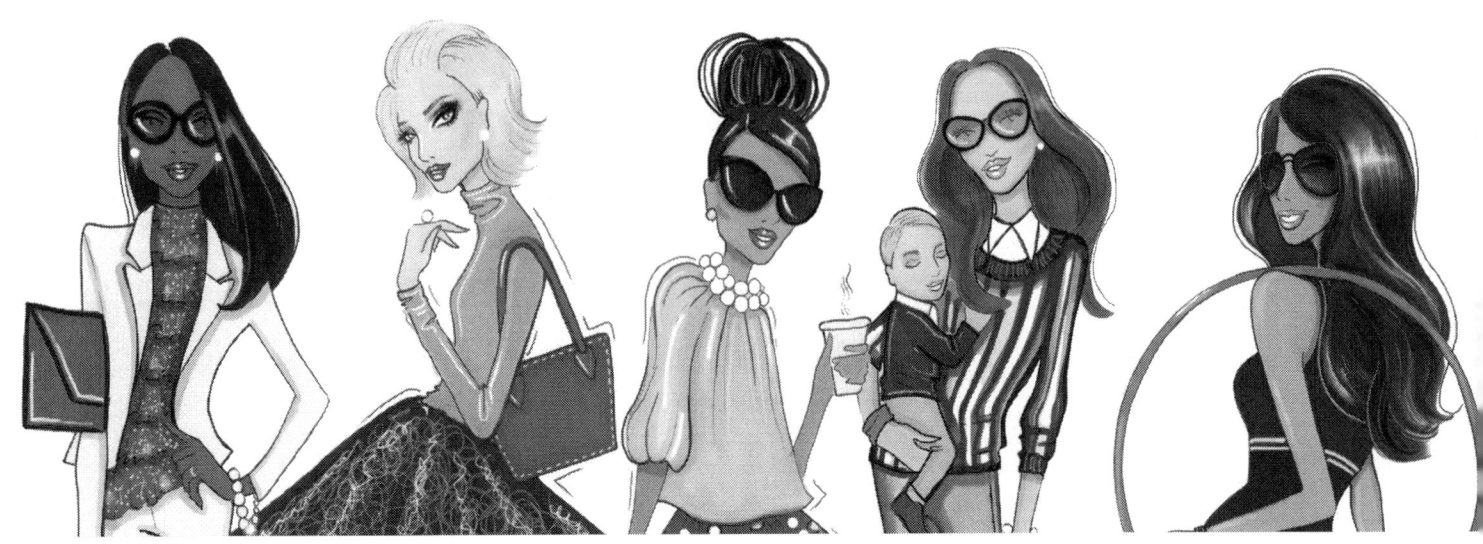

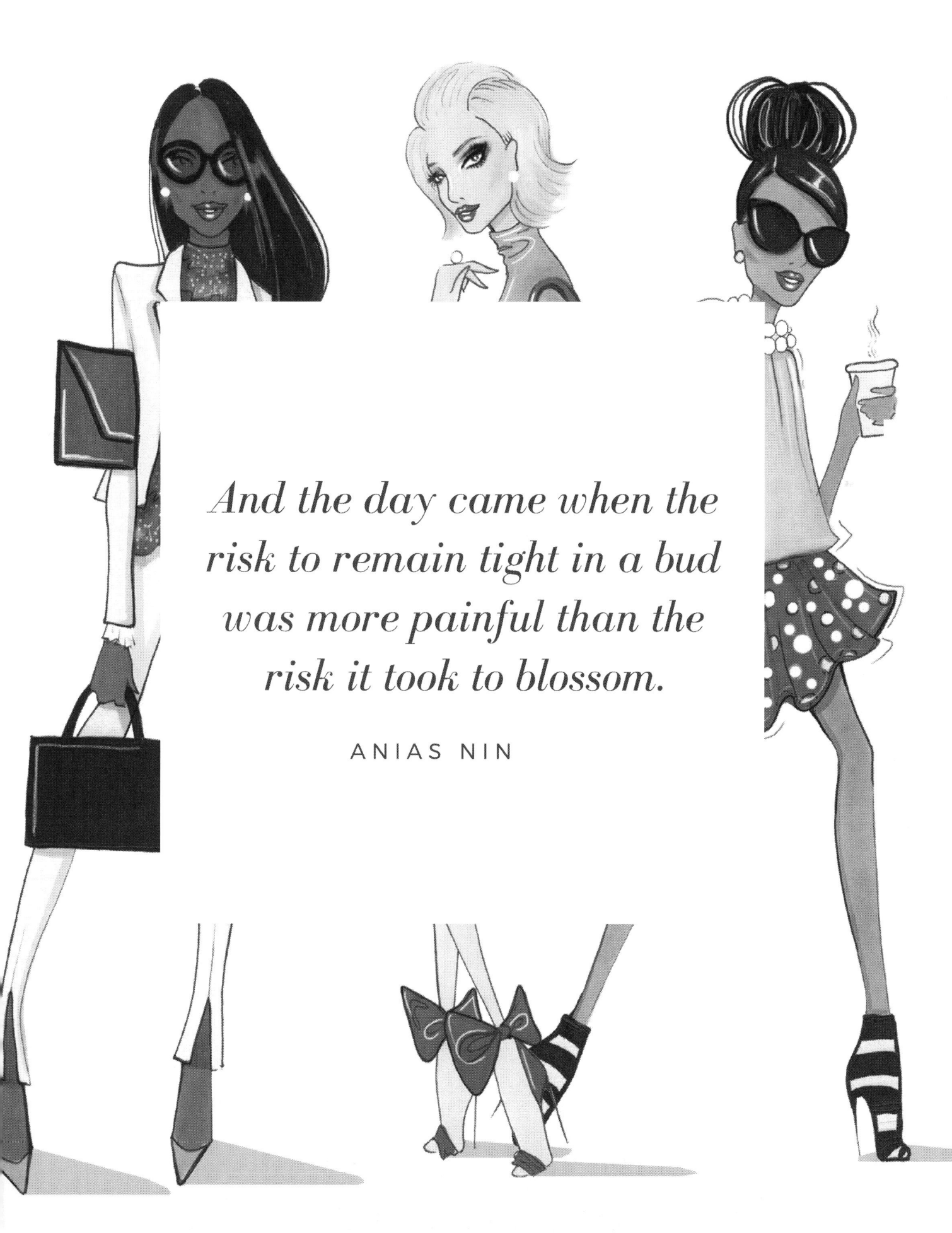

And the day came when the risk to remain tight in a bud was more painful than the risk it took to blossom.

ANIAS NIN

The blessing is in the execution!

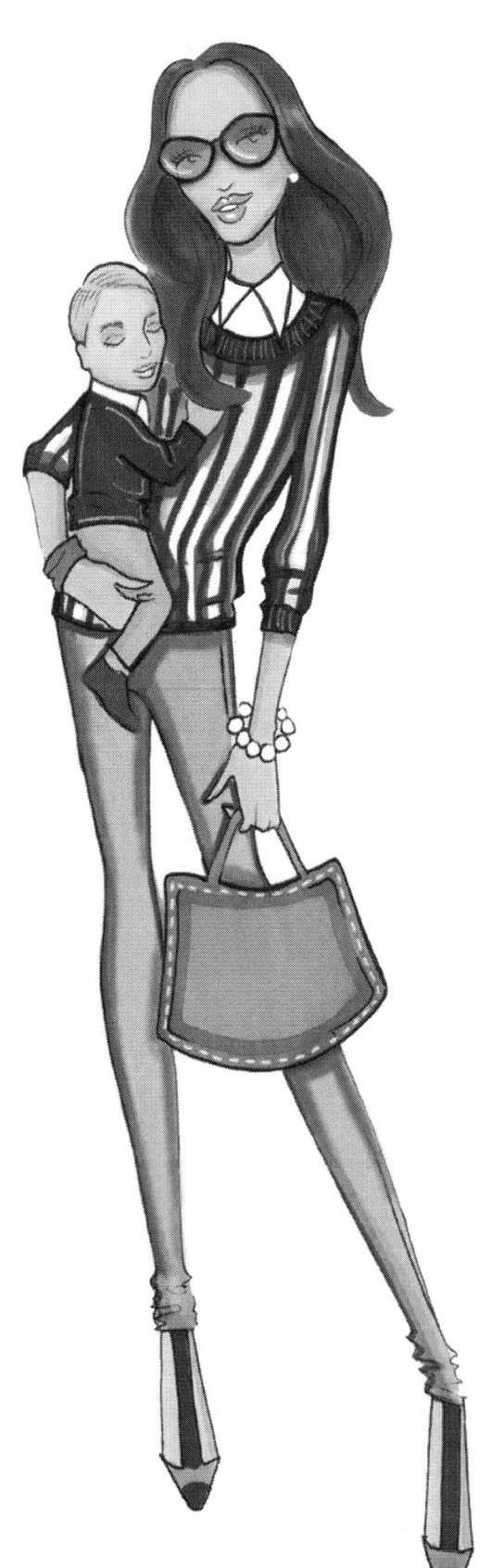

Let's go back to our theme Scripture, Isaiah 32:8.

"But the noble make noble plans and by noble deeds they stand."

Now that you've made your noble plan, it's time to put noble deeds behind it.

Start your day by filling out "Your 5."

1. Pick the ONE most important thing that will move your life/business/project forward that day.

2. Remind yourself of the goal this applies to.

3. Get yourself focused on your strengths instead of your weaknesses right away.

4. Stop your negative self-talk before it starts.

5. Commit to filling up after a day of pouring out.

Then list the rest of your to-do's for the day and set your mind on gratitude instead of scarcity.

Reference the quote at the top of each page for encouragement throughout the day.

Commit to this routine every morning, and you'll be on your way to a happier you!

I have come that they may have life, and have it to the full. - John 10:10

Design your happy. With God. On Purpose.

Date: _____

Every expert was once a beginner. The key is to begin.
- Helen Hayes

The one thing I'll accomplish to win today is:
_____
_____

The life goal this applies to is:
_____
_____

The skills and talents I will use to do this are:
_____
_____

An empowering thought to help is:
_____
_____

My self-care action for today is:
_____
_____

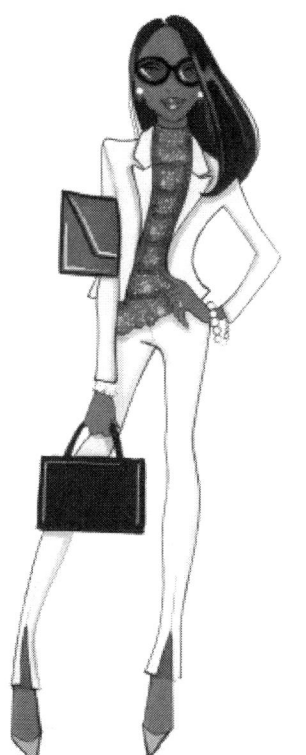

Other To-Do's:	Today I'm thankful for:

Design Your Happy. With God. On Purpose.

Date: _____

I'm always perpetually out of my comfort zone.
- Tory Burch

The one thing I'll accomplish to win today is:
_____
_____

The life goal this applies to is:
_____
_____

The skills and talents I will use to do this are:
_____
_____

An empowering thought to help is:
_____
_____

My self-care action for today is:
_____
_____

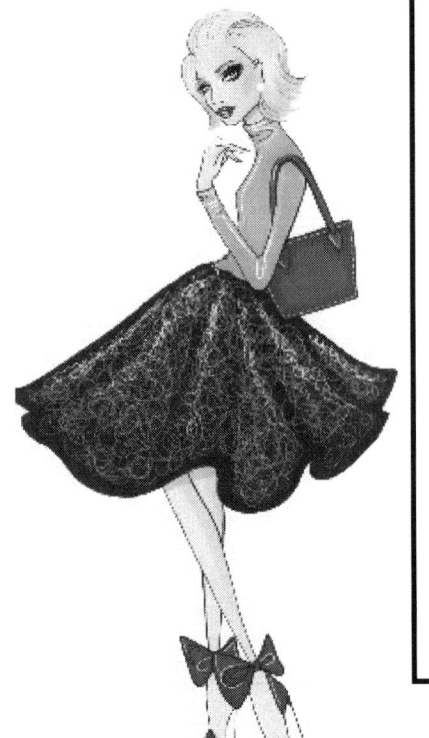

Other To-Do's:	Today I'm thankful for:

Design Your Happy. With God. On Purpose.

Date: _____

Give thanks to the Lord, for He is good.
- Psalm 136:1

The one thing I'll accomplish to win today is:
_____
_____

The life goal this applies to is:
_____
_____

The skills and talents I will use to do this are:
_____
_____

An empowering thought to help is:
_____
_____

My self-care action for today is:
_____
_____

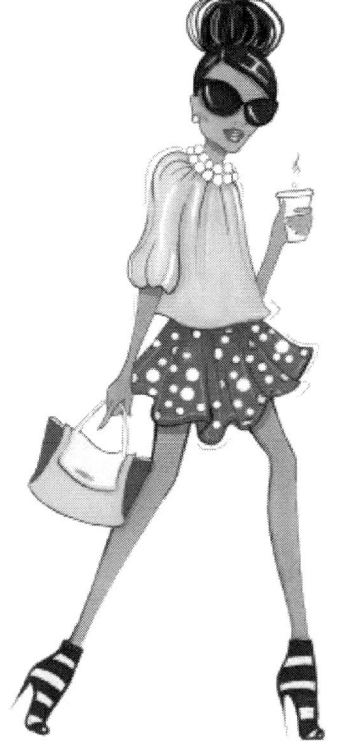

Other To-Do's:	Today I'm thankful for:

Design Your Happy. With God. On Purpose.

Date: _____

Action expresses priorities.
- Gandhi

The one thing I'll accomplish to win today is:
_____
_____

The life goal this applies to is:
_____
_____

The skills and talents I will use to do this are:
_____
_____

An empowering thought to help is:
_____
_____

My self-care action for today is:
_____
_____

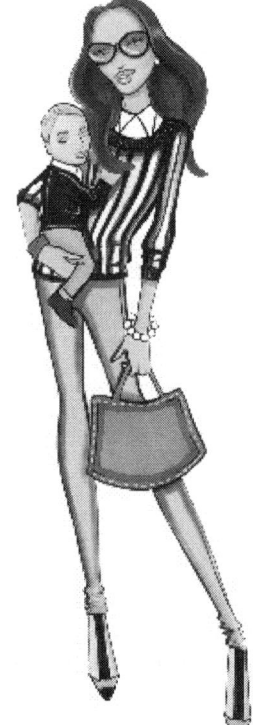

Other To-Do's:	Today I'm thankful for:

Design Your Happy. With God. On Purpose.

Date: _____

If you haven't felt like quitting, your dreams aren't big enough.
- Kelly Osbourn

The one thing I'll accomplish to win today is:
_____
_____

The life goal this applies to is:
_____
_____

The skills and talents I will use to do this are:
_____
_____

An empowering thought to help is:
_____
_____

My self-care action for today is:
_____
_____

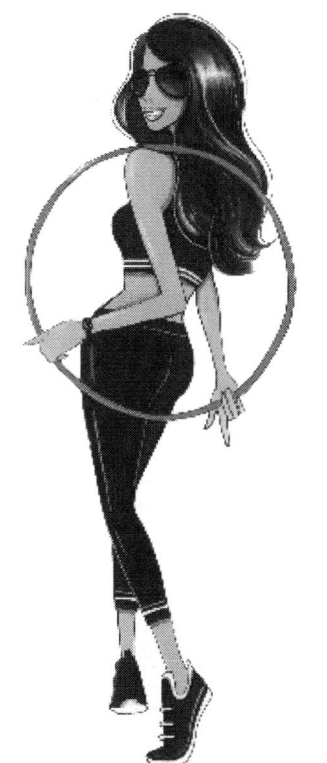

Other To-Do's:	Today I'm thankful for:

Design Your Happy. With God. On Purpose.

Date: _____

Everyone shines, given the right lighting.
- Susan Cain

The one thing I'll accomplish to win today is:
_____
_____

The life goal this applies to is:
_____
_____

The skills and talents I will use to do this are:
_____
_____

An empowering thought to help is:
_____
_____

My self-care action for today is:
_____
_____

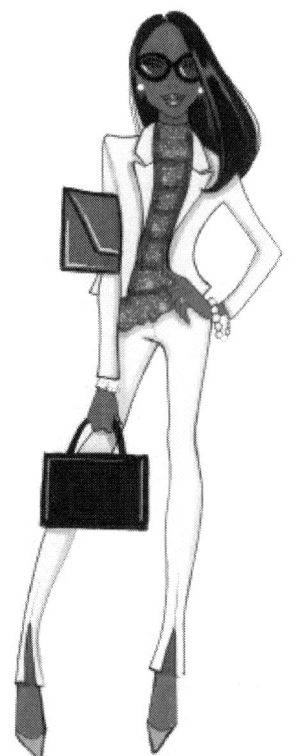

Other To-Do's:	Today I'm thankful for:

Design Your Happy. With God. On Purpose.

Date: _____

The challenge is not to be perfect. It's to be whole.
- Jane Fonda

The one thing I'll accomplish to win today is:
_____
_____

The life goal this applies to is:
_____
_____

The skills and talents I will use to do this are:
_____
_____

An empowering thought to help is:
_____
_____

My self-care action for today is:
_____
_____

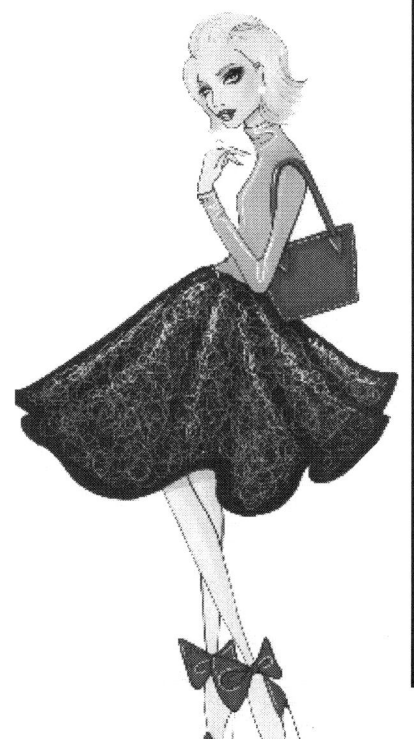

Other To-Do's:	Today I'm thankful for:

Design Your Happy. With God. On Purpose.

Date: _____

The ceiling of confidence is the floor of faith.
- Chantelle Anderson

The one thing I'll accomplish to win today is:
_____
_____

The life goal this applies to is:
_____
_____

The skills and talents I will use to do this are:
_____
_____

An empowering thought to help is:
_____
_____

My self-care action for today is:
_____
_____

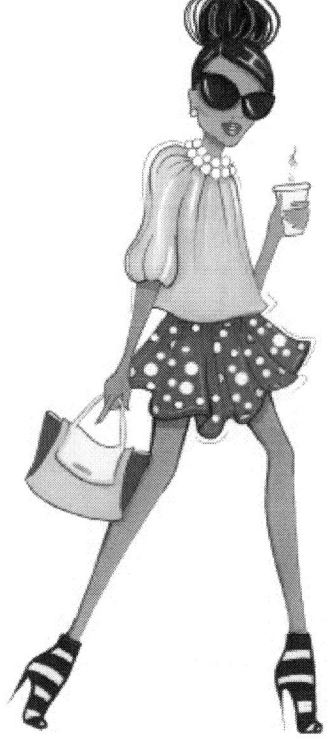

Other To-Do's:	Today I'm thankful for:

Design Your Happy. With God. On Purpose.

Date: _____

Do one thing every day that scares you.
- Eleanor Roosevelt

The one thing I'll accomplish to win today is:
_____
_____

The life goal this applies to is:
_____
_____

The skills and talents I will use to do this are:
_____
_____

An empowering thought to help is:
_____
_____

My self-care action for today is:
_____
_____

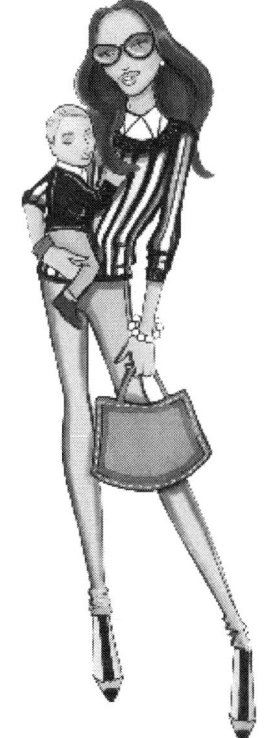

Other To-Do's:	Today I'm thankful for:

Design Your Happy. With God. On Purpose.

Date: _____

I believe happy girls are the prettiest girls.
- Audrey Hepburn

The one thing I'll accomplish to win today is:
_____
_____

The life goal this applies to is:
_____
_____

The skills and talents I will use to do this are:
_____
_____

An empowering thought to help is:
_____
_____

My self-care action for today is:
_____
_____

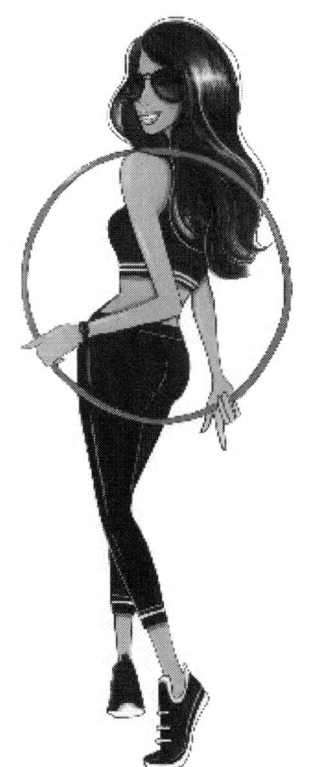

Other To-Do's:	Today I'm thankful for:

Design Your Happy. With God. On Purpose.

Date: _____

Identify the most relevant actions and do them very well.
- Kim Feil

The one thing I'll accomplish to win today is:
_____
_____

The life goal this applies to is:
_____
_____

The skills and talents I will use to do this are:
_____
_____

An empowering thought to help is:
_____
_____

My self-care action for today is:
_____
_____

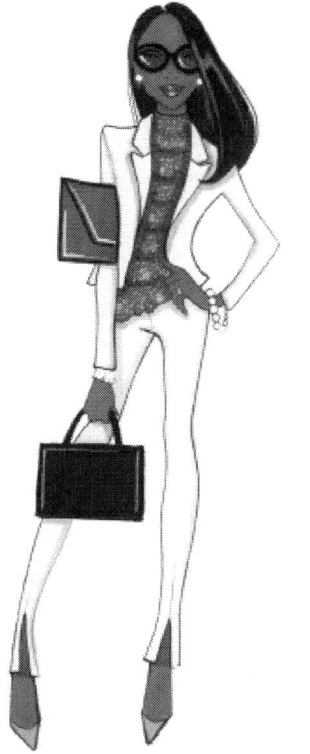

Other To-Do's:	Today I'm thankful for:

Design Your Happy. With God. On Purpose.

Date: _____

Your Word is a lamp for my feet, a light on my path.
- Psalm 119:105

The one thing I'll accomplish to win today is:
_____
_____

The life goal this applies to is:
_____
_____

The skills and talents I will use to do this are:
_____
_____

An empowering thought to help is:
_____
_____

My self-care action for today is:
_____
_____

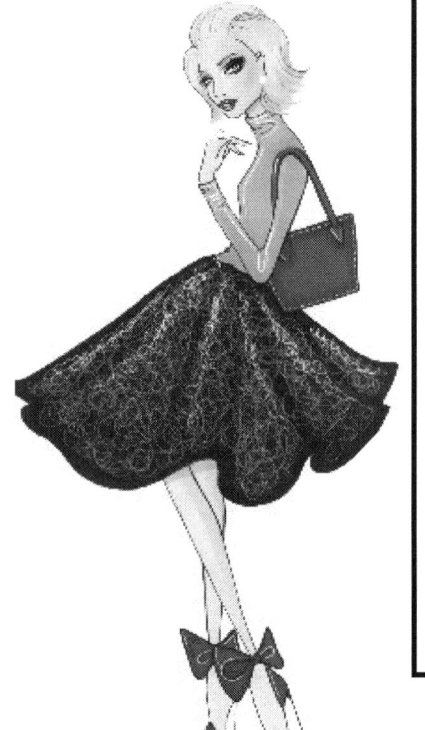

Other To-Do's:	Today I'm thankful for:

Design Your Happy. With God. On Purpose.

Date: _____

Take criticism seriously but not personally.
- Hillary Clinton

The one thing I'll accomplish to win today is:
_____
_____

The life goal this applies to is:
_____
_____

The skills and talents I will use to do this are:
_____
_____

An empowering thought to help is:
_____
_____

My self-care action for today is:
_____
_____

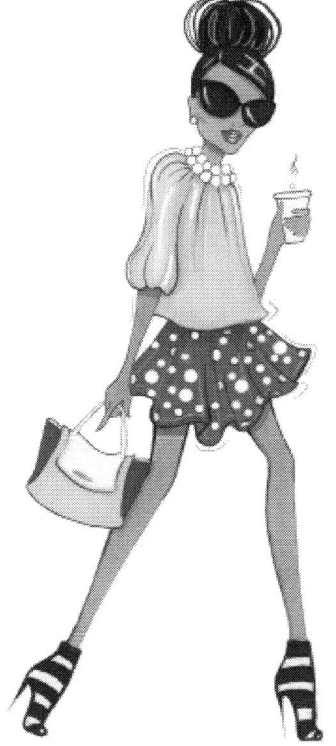

Other To-Do's:	Today I'm thankful for:

Design Your Happy. With God. On Purpose.

Date: _____

Because your love is better than life, my lips will glorify you.
- Psalm 63:3

The one thing I'll accomplish to win today is:
_____
_____

The life goal this applies to is:
_____
_____

The skills and talents I will use to do this are:
_____
_____

An empowering thought to help is:
_____
_____

My self-care action for today is:
_____
_____

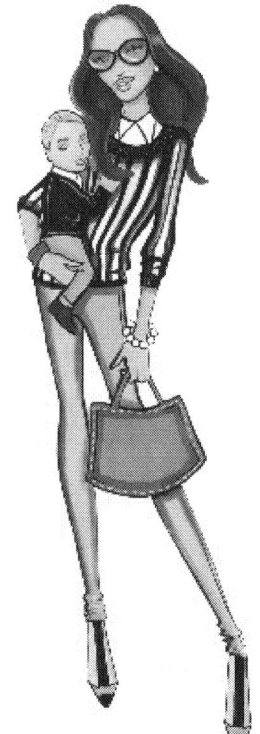

Other To-Do's:	Today I'm thankful for:

Design Your Happy. With God. On Purpose.

Date: _____

The most courageous act is still to think for yourself. Aloud.
- Coco Chanel

The one thing I'll accomplish to win today is:
___
___

The life goal this applies to is:
___
___

The skills and talents I will use to do this are:
___
___

An empowering thought to help is:
___
___

My self-care action for today is:
___
___

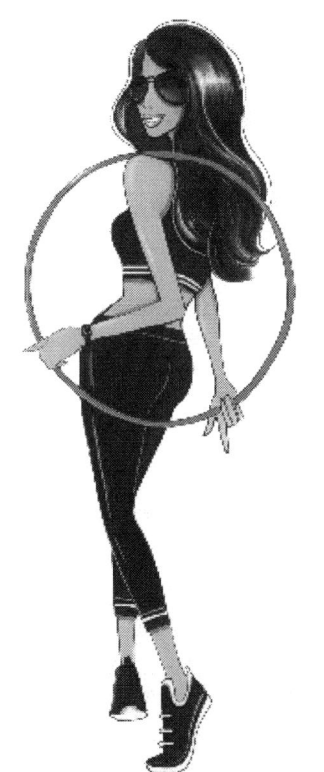

Other To-Do's:	Today I'm thankful for:

Design Your Happy. With God. On Purpose.

Date: _____

You may have to fight a battle more than once to win.
- Margaret Thatcher

The one thing I'll accomplish to win today is:
_____
_____

The life goal this applies to is:
_____
_____

The skills and talents I will use to do this are:
_____
_____

An empowering thought to help is:
_____
_____

My self-care action for today is:
_____
_____

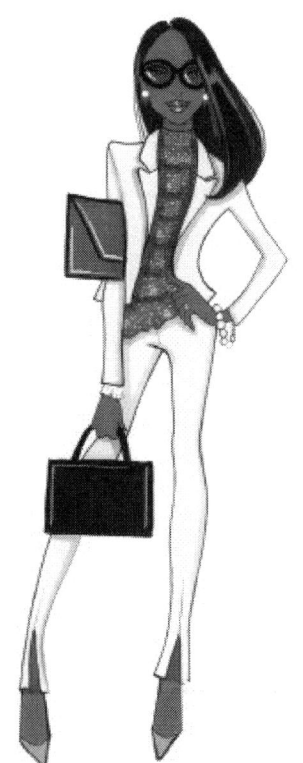

Other To-Do's:	Today I'm thankful for:

Design Your Happy. With God. On Purpose.

Date: _____

The only way to do great work is to do what you love.
- Steve Jobs

The one thing I'll accomplish to win today is:
_____
_____

The life goal this applies to is:
_____
_____

The skills and talents I will use to do this are:
_____
_____

An empowering thought to help is:
_____
_____

My self-care action for today is:
_____
_____

Other To-Do's:	Today I'm thankful for:

Design Your Happy. With God. On Purpose.

Date: _____

The way you tell your story to yourself matters.
- Amy Cuddy

The one thing I'll accomplish to win today is:
_____
_____

The life goal this applies to is:
_____
_____

The skills and talents I will use to do this are:
_____
_____

An empowering thought to help is:
_____
_____

My self-care action for today is:
_____
_____

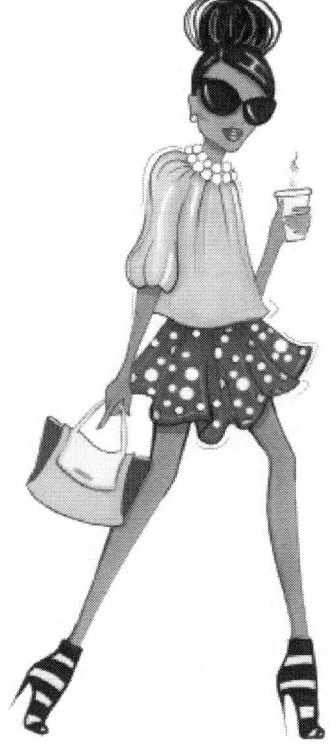

Other To-Do's:	Today I'm thankful for:

Design Your Happy. With God. On Purpose.

Date: _____

Find out who you are and do it on purpose.
- Dolly Parton

The one thing I'll accomplish to win today is:
_____
_____

The life goal this applies to is:
_____
_____

The skills and talents I will use to do this are:
_____
_____

An empowering thought to help is:
_____
_____

My self-care action for today is:
_____
_____

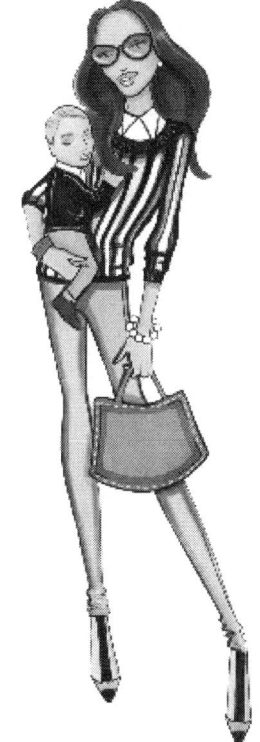

Other To-Do's:	Today I'm thankful for:

Design Your Happy. With God. On Purpose.

Date: _____

You must do the thing you think you cannot do.
- Eleanor Roosevelt

The one thing I'll accomplish to win today is:
_____
_____

The life goal this applies to is:
_____
_____

The skills and talents I will use to do this are:
_____
_____

An empowering thought to help is:
_____
_____

My self-care action for today is:
_____
_____

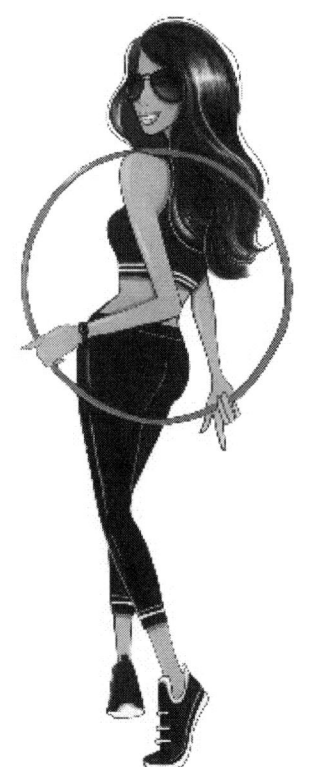

Other To-Do's:	Today I'm thankful for:

Design Your Happy. With God. On Purpose.

Date: _____

When I let go of what I am, I become what I might be.
- Lao Tzu

The one thing I'll accomplish to win today is:
_____
_____

The life goal this applies to is:
_____
_____

The skills and talents I will use to do this are:
_____
_____

An empowering thought to help is:
_____
_____

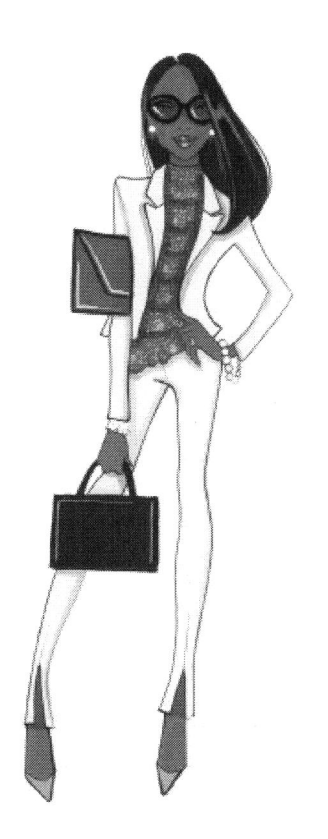

My self-care action for today is:
_____
_____

Other To-Do's:	Today I'm thankful for:

Design Your Happy. With God. On Purpose.

Date: _____

Dreaming, after all, is a form of planning.
- Gloria Steinem

The one thing I'll accomplish to win today is:
_____
_____

The life goal this applies to is:
_____
_____

The skills and talents I will use to do this are:
_____
_____

An empowering thought to help is:
_____
_____

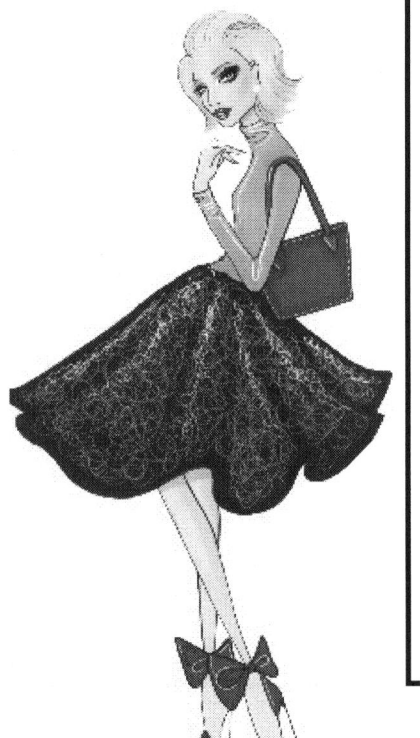

My self-care action for today is:
_____
_____

Other To-Do's:	Today I'm thankful for:

Design Your Happy. With God. On Purpose.

Date: _____

Victory is won through many advisors.
- Proverbs 11:14

The one thing I'll accomplish to win today is:
_____
_____

The life goal this applies to is:
_____
_____

The skills and talents I will use to do this are:
_____
_____

An empowering thought to help is:
_____
_____

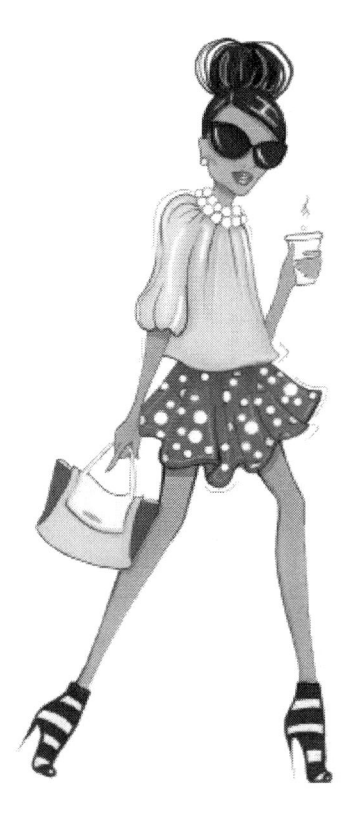

My self-care action for today is:
_____
_____

Other To-Do's:	Today I'm thankful for:

Design Your Happy. With God. On Purpose.

Date: _____

Write something worth reading or do something worth writing.
- Ben Franklin

The one thing I'll accomplish to win today is:
_____
_____

The life goal this applies to is:
_____
_____

The skills and talents I will use to do this are:
_____
_____

An empowering thought to help is:
_____
_____

My self-care action for today is:
_____
_____

Other To-Do's:	Today I'm thankful for:

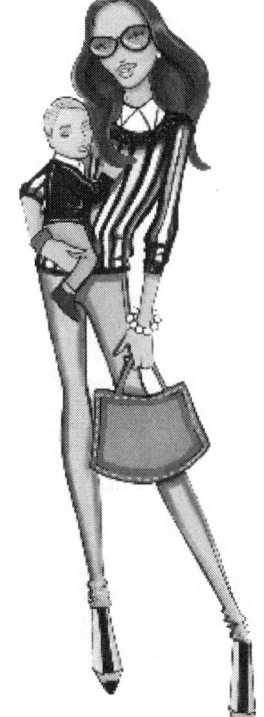

Design Your Happy. With God. On Purpose.

Date: _____

Amazing how we can light tomorrow with today.
- Elizabeth Browning

The one thing I'll accomplish to win today is:
_____
_____

The life goal this applies to is:
_____
_____

The skills and talents I will use to do this are:
_____
_____

An empowering thought to help is:
_____
_____

My self-care action for today is:
_____
_____

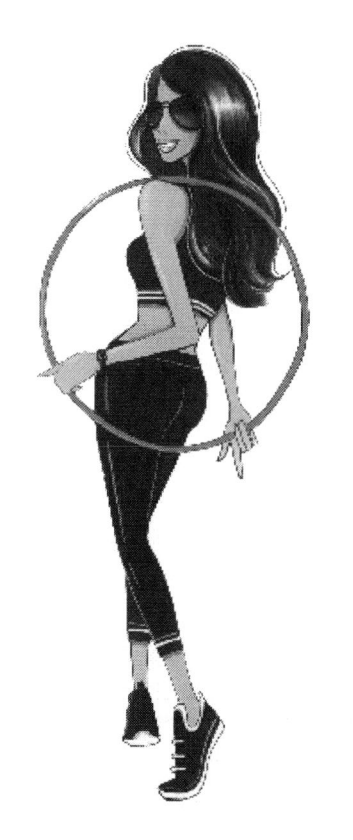

Other To-Do's:	Today I'm thankful for:

Design Your Happy. With God. On Purpose.

Date: _____

It is never too late to be what you might have been.
- George Eliot

The one thing I'll accomplish to win today is:
_____
_____

The life goal this applies to is:
_____
_____

The skills and talents I will use to do this are:
_____
_____

An empowering thought to help is:
_____
_____

My self-care action for today is:
_____
_____

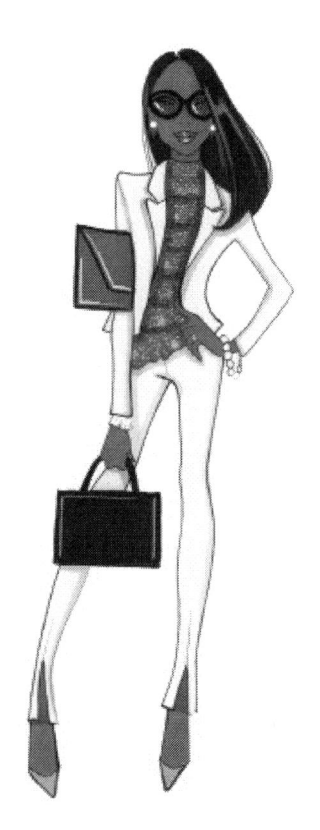

Other To-Do's:	Today I'm thankful for:

Design Your Happy. With God. On Purpose.

Date: _____

Charisma is public self-acceptance.
- Unkown

The one thing I'll accomplish to win today is:
_____
_____

The life goal this applies to is:
_____
_____

The skills and talents I will use to do this are:
_____
_____

An empowering thought to help is:
_____
_____

My self-care action for today is:
_____
_____

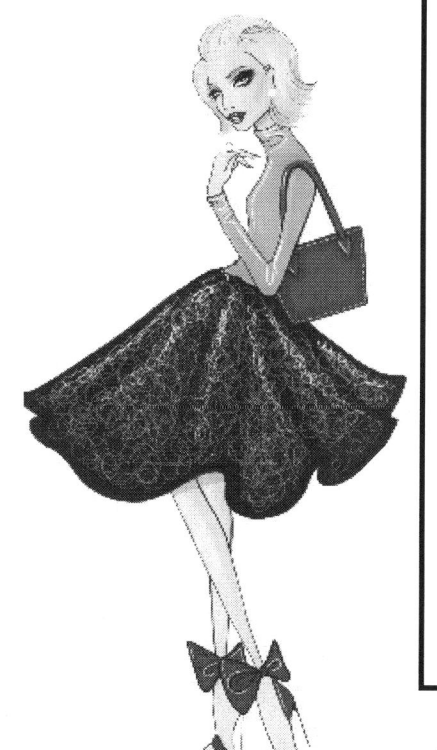

Other To-Do's:	Today I'm thankful for:

Design Your Happy. With God. On Purpose.

Date: _____

You can't think crooked and walk straight.
- Anon

The one thing I'll accomplish to win today is:
_____
_____

The life goal this applies to is:
_____
_____

The skills and talents I will use to do this are:
_____
_____

An empowering thought to help is:
_____
_____

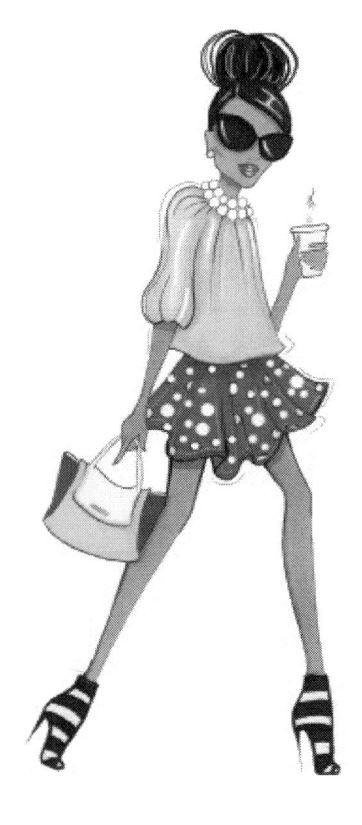

My self-care action for today is:
_____
_____

Other To-Do's:	Today I'm thankful for:

Design Your Happy. With God. On Purpose.

Date: _____

Better a diamond with a flaw than a pebble without one.
- Chinese Proverb

The one thing I'll accomplish to win today is:
_____
_____

The life goal this applies to is:
_____
_____

The skills and talents I will use to do this are:
_____
_____

An empowering thought to help is:
_____
_____

My self-care action for today is:
_____
_____

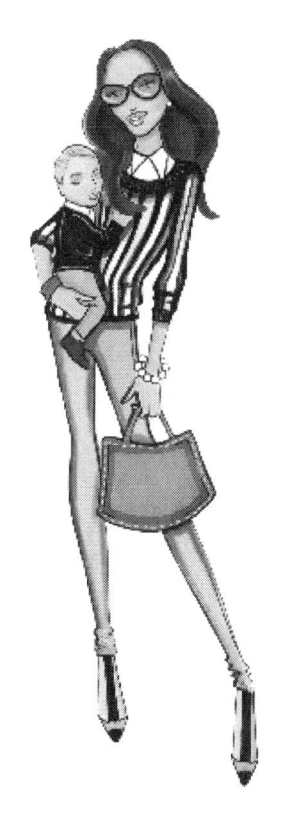

Other To-Do's:	Today I'm thankful for:

Design Your Happy. With God. On Purpose.

Date: _____

What would you do if you knew you could not fail?
- Jeff Goins

The one thing I'll accomplish to win today is:
_____
_____

The life goal this applies to is:
_____
_____

The skills and talents I will use to do this are:
_____
_____

An empowering thought to help is:
_____
_____

My self-care action for today is:
_____
_____

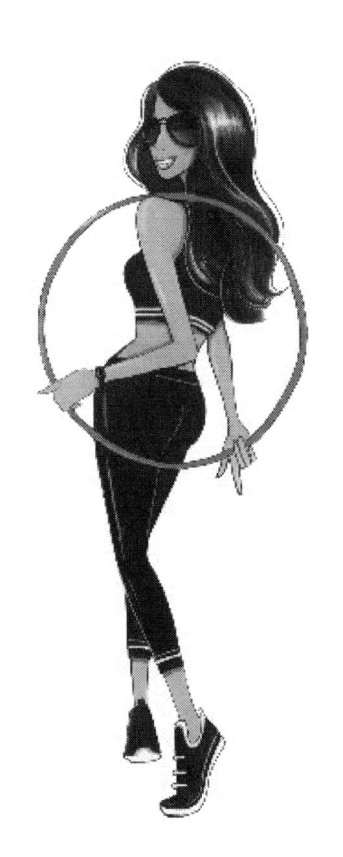

Other To-Do's:

Today I'm thankful for:

Design Your Happy. With God. On Purpose.

Date: _____

Well done is better than well said.
- Benjamin Franklin

The one thing I'll accomplish to win today is:
_____
_____

The life goal this applies to is:
_____
_____

The skills and talents I will use to do this are:
_____
_____

An empowering thought to help is:
_____
_____

My self-care action for today is:
_____
_____

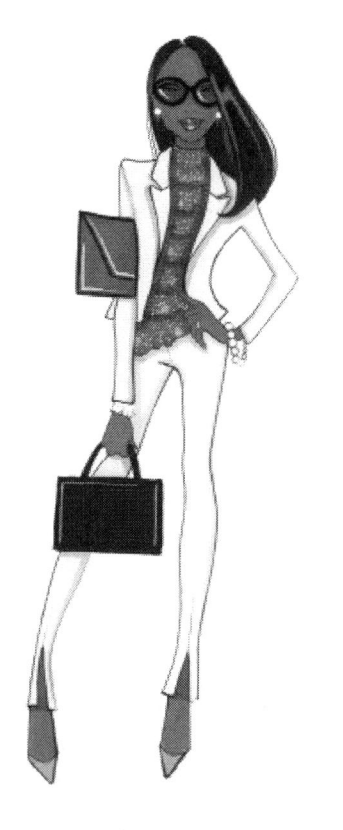

Other To-Do's:	Today I'm thankful for:

Design Your Happy. With God. On Purpose.

Date: _____

Diligent hands will rule but laziness ends in forced labor.
- Proverbs 12:24

The one thing I'll accomplish to win today is:
_____
_____

The life goal this applies to is:
_____
_____

The skills and talents I will use to do this are:
_____
_____

An empowering thought to help is:
_____
_____

My self-care action for today is:
_____
_____

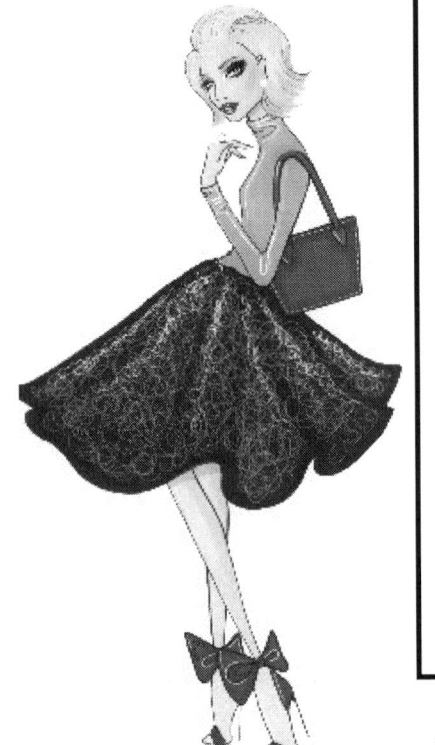

Other To-Do's:	Today I'm thankful for:

Design Your Happy. With God. On Purpose.

Date: _____

I am the way, the truth and the life.
- Jesus (John 14:6)

The one thing I'll accomplish to win today is:
_____
_____

The life goal this applies to is:
_____
_____

The skills and talents I will use to do this are:
_____
_____

An empowering thought to help is:
_____
_____

My self-care action for today is:
_____
_____

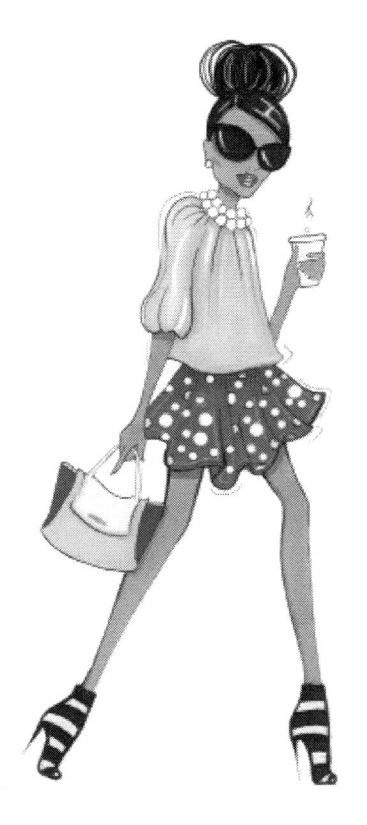

Other To-Do's:	Today I'm thankful for:

Design Your Happy. With God. On Purpose.

Date: _____

The further I get, the further I want to go.
- Nas

The one thing I'll accomplish to win today is:
_____
_____

The life goal this applies to is:
_____
_____

The skills and talents I will use to do this are:
_____
_____

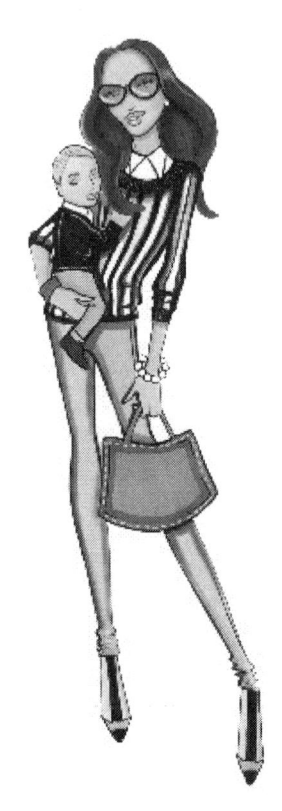

An empowering thought to help is:
_____
_____

My self-care action for today is:
_____
_____

Other To-Do's:	Today I'm thankful for:

Design Your Happy. With God. On Purpose.

Date: _____

We have this huge collective power - if only we'd use it.
- Jane Goodall

The one thing I'll accomplish to win today is:
_____
_____

The life goal this applies to is:
_____
_____

The skills and talents I will use to do this are:
_____
_____

An empowering thought to help is:
_____
_____

My self-care action for today is:
_____
_____

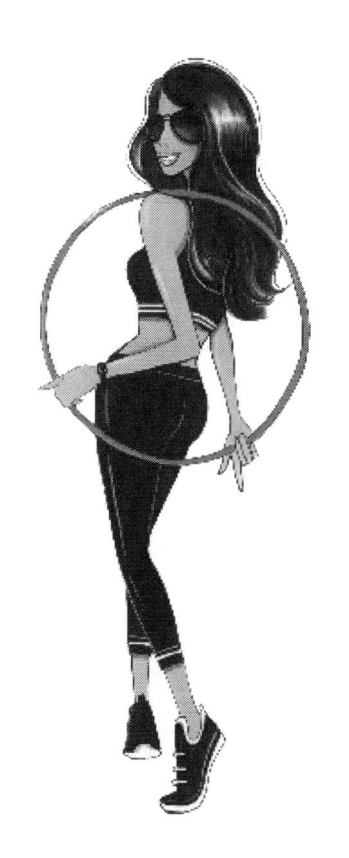

Other To-Do's:	Today I'm thankful for:

Design Your Happy. With God. On Purpose.

Date: _____

Peacemakers who sow in peace reap a harvest of righteousness.
- James 3:18

The one thing I'll accomplish to win today is:
_____
_____

The life goal this applies to is:
_____
_____

The skills and talents I will use to do this are:
_____
_____

An empowering thought to help is:
_____
_____

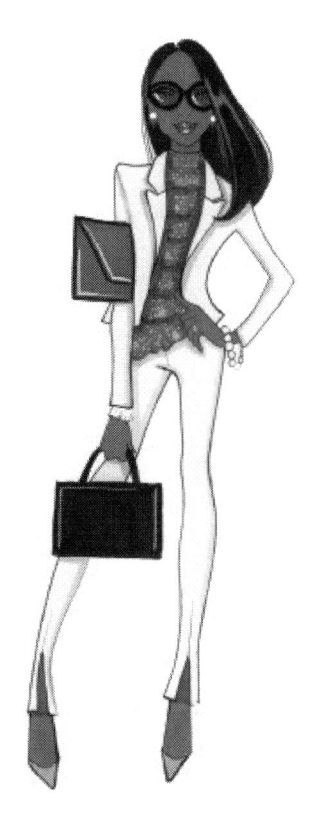

My self-care action for today is:
_____
_____

Other To-Do's:	Today I'm thankful for:

Design Your Happy. With God. On Purpose.

Date: _____

What we have to learn to do, we learn by doing.
- Aristotle

The one thing I'll accomplish to win today is:
_____
_____

The life goal this applies to is:
_____
_____

The skills and talents I will use to do this are:
_____
_____

An empowering thought to help is:
_____
_____

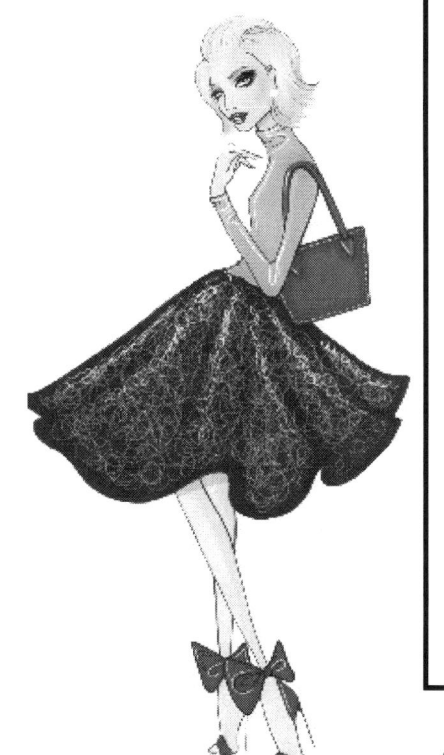

My self-care action for today is:
_____
_____

Other To-Do's:	Today I'm thankful for:

Design Your Happy. With God. On Purpose.

Date: _____

Each experience enables the next one.
- Marie Quintana

The one thing I'll accomplish to win today is:
_____
_____

The life goal this applies to is:
_____
_____

The skills and talents I will use to do this are:
_____
_____

An empowering thought to help is:
_____
_____

My self-care action for today is:
_____
_____

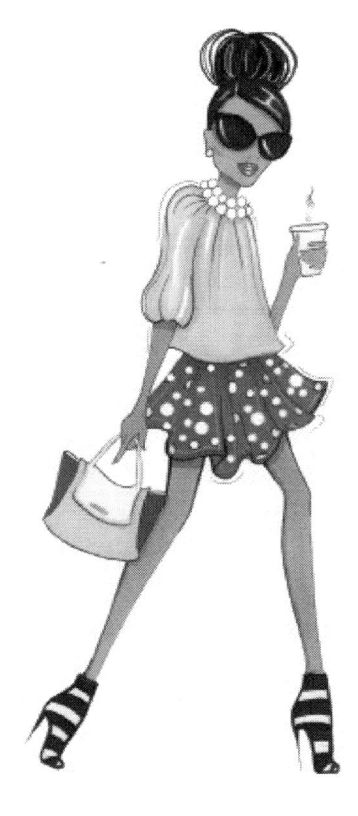

Other To-Do's:	Today I'm thankful for:

Design Your Happy. With God. On Purpose.

Date: _____

For though the righteous fall seven times, they rise again.
- Proverbs 24:16

The one thing I'll accomplish to win today is:
_____
_____

The life goal this applies to is:
_____
_____

The skills and talents I will use to do this are:
_____
_____

An empowering thought to help is:
_____
_____

My self-care action for today is:
_____
_____

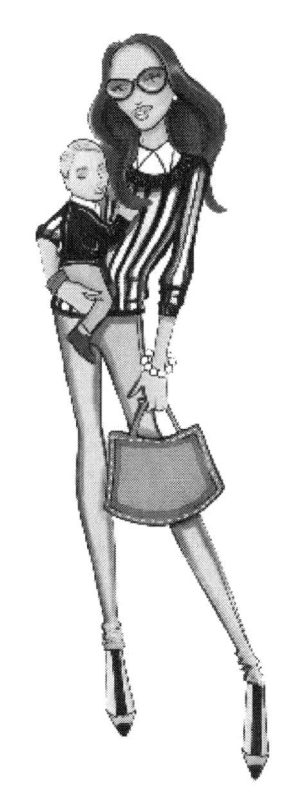

Other To-Do's:	Today I'm thankful for:

Design Your Happy. With God. On Purpose.

Date: _____

My grace is sufficient...for my power is made perfect in weakness.
- 2 Corinthians 12:9

The one thing I'll accomplish to win today is:
_____
_____

The life goal this applies to is:
_____
_____

The skills and talents I will use to do this are:
_____
_____

An empowering thought to help is:
_____
_____

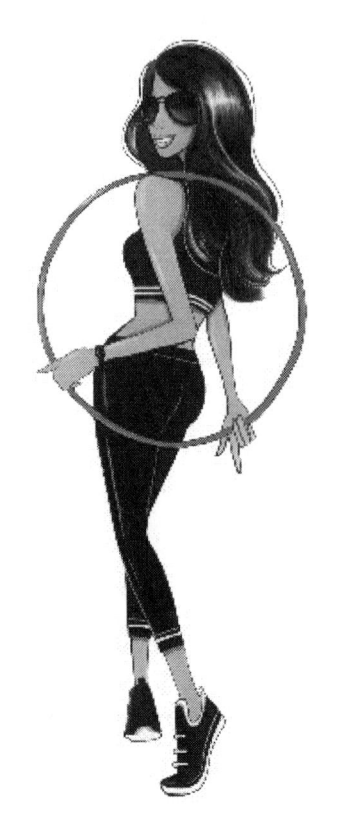

My self-care action for today is:
_____
_____

Other To-Do's:	Today I'm thankful for:

Design Your Happy. With God. On Purpose.

Date: _____

At the end of the day, you have to like yourself.
- Martina Navratilova

The one thing I'll accomplish to win today is:
_____
_____

The life goal this applies to is:
_____
_____

The skills and talents I will use to do this are:
_____
_____

An empowering thought to help is:
_____
_____

My self-care action for today is:
_____
_____

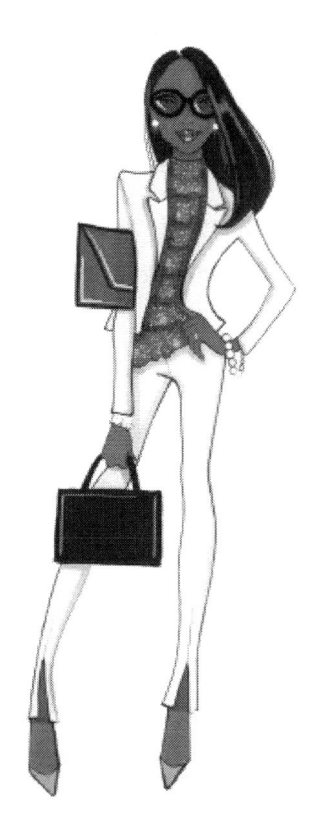

Other To-Do's:	Today I'm thankful for:

Design Your Happy. With God. On Purpose.

Date: _____

All that matters is love and work.
- Sigmund Freud

The one thing I'll accomplish to win today is:
_____
_____

The life goal this applies to is:
_____
_____

The skills and talents I will use to do this are:
_____
_____

An empowering thought to help is:
_____
_____

My self-care action for today is:
_____
_____

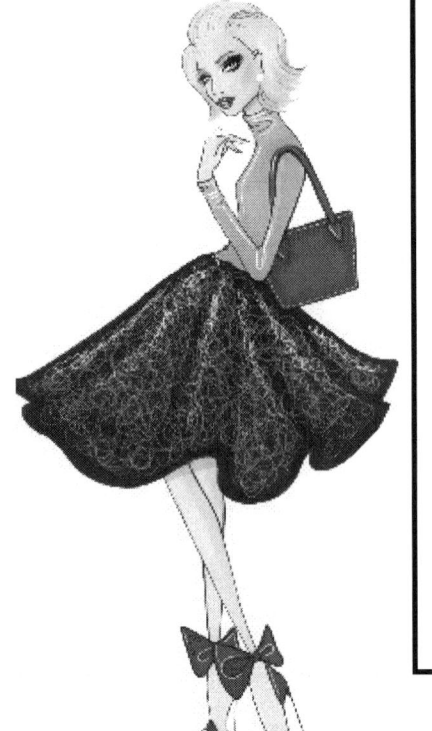

Other To-Do's:	Today I'm thankful for:

Design Your Happy. With God. On Purpose.

Date: _____

Anything that is not love is a cry for it.
- Unknown

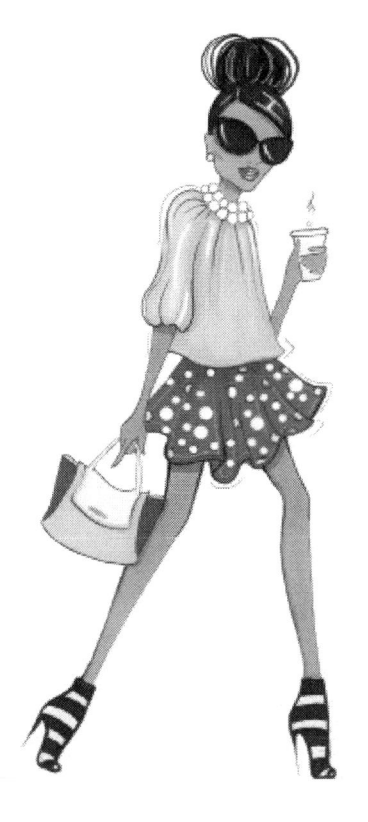

The one thing I'll accomplish to win today is:
_____
_____

The life goal this applies to is:
_____
_____

The skills and talents I will use to do this are:
_____
_____

An empowering thought to help is:
_____
_____

My self-care action for today is:
_____
_____

Other To-Do's:	Today I'm thankful for:

Design Your Happy. With God. On Purpose.

Date: _____

Risk is a choice. It is the only way to test your potential.
- Sylvia Earle

The one thing I'll accomplish to win today is:
_____
_____

The life goal this applies to is:
_____
_____

The skills and talents I will use to do this are:
_____
_____

An empowering thought to help is:
_____
_____

My self-care action for today is:
_____
_____

Other To-Do's:	Today I'm thankful for:

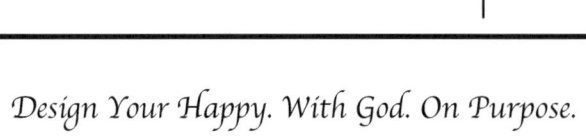

Design Your Happy. With God. On Purpose.

Date: _____

The Lord makes firm the steps of the one who delights in Him.
- Psalm 37:23

The one thing I'll accomplish to win today is:
_____
_____

The life goal this applies to is:
_____
_____

The skills and talents I will use to do this are:
_____
_____

An empowering thought to help is:
_____
_____

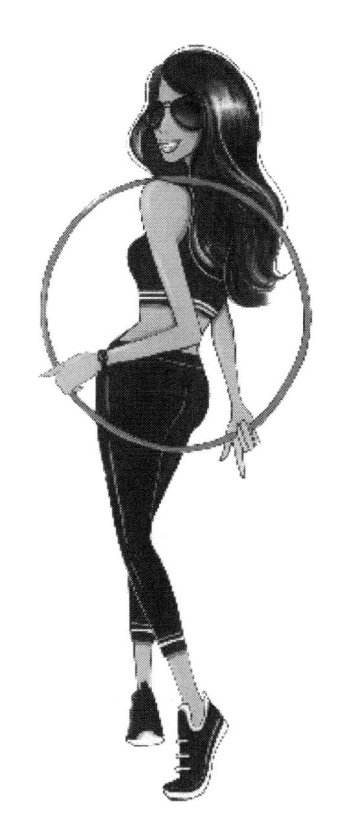

My self-care action for today is:
_____
_____

Other To-Do's:	Today I'm thankful for:

Design Your Happy. With God. On Purpose.

Date: _____

Wealth is the ability to fully experience life.
- Henry David Thoreau

The one thing I'll accomplish to win today is:
_____
_____

The life goal this applies to is:
_____
_____

The skills and talents I will use to do this are:
_____
_____

An empowering thought to help is:
_____
_____

My self-care action for today is:
_____
_____

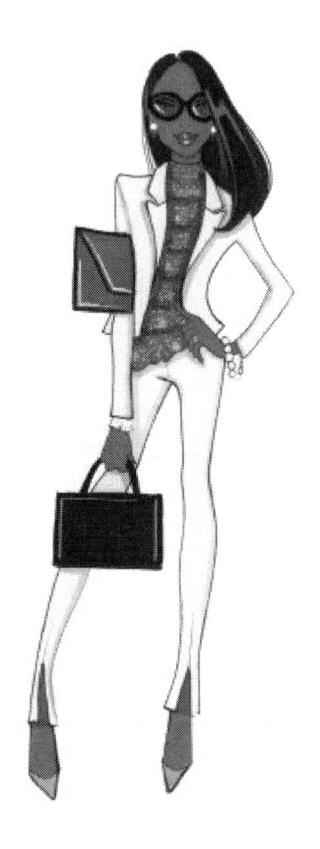

Other To-Do's:	Today I'm thankful for:

Design Your Happy. With God. On Purpose.

Date: _____

Nothing great was ever achieved without enthusiasm.
- Ralph Waldo Emerson

The one thing I'll accomplish to win today is:
_____
_____

The life goal this applies to is:
_____
_____

The skills and talents I will use to do this are:
_____
_____

An empowering thought to help is:
_____
_____

My self-care action for today is:
_____
_____

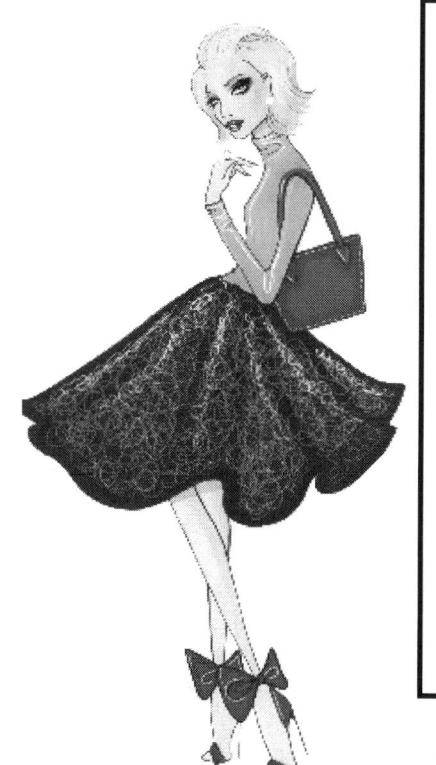

Other To-Do's:	Today I'm thankful for:

Design Your Happy. With God. On Purpose.

Date: _____

You have to lose some battles in order to win the war.
- Alex Sink

The one thing I'll accomplish to win today is:
_____
_____

The life goal this applies to is:
_____
_____

The skills and talents I will use to do this are:
_____
_____

An empowering thought to help is:
_____
_____

My self-care action for today is:
_____
_____

Other To-Do's:	Today I'm thankful for:

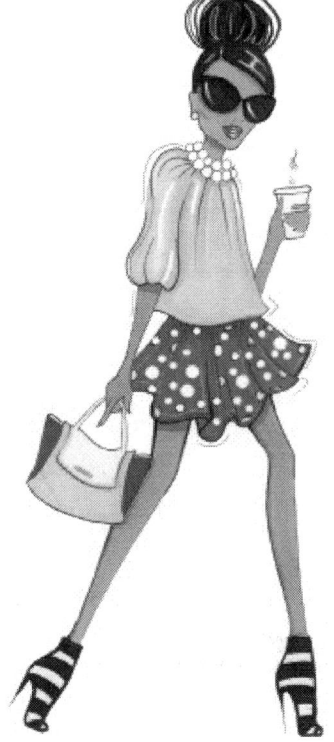

Design Your Happy. With God. On Purpose.

Date: _____

The mind is not a vessel to be filled but a fire to be kindled.
- Plutarch

The one thing I'll accomplish to win today is:
_____
_____

The life goal this applies to is:
_____
_____

The skills and talents I will use to do this are:
_____
_____

An empowering thought to help is:
_____
_____

My self-care action for today is:
_____
_____

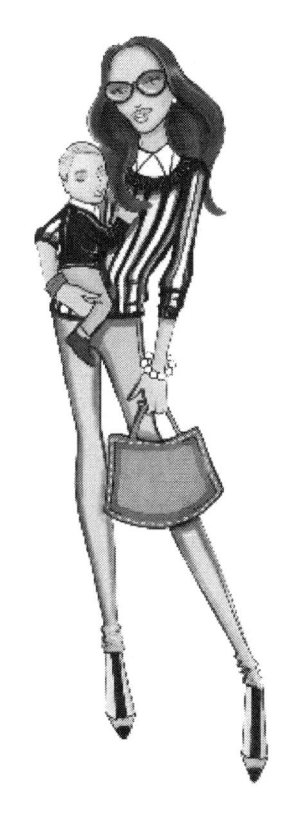

Other To-Do's:	Today I'm thankful for:

Design Your Happy. With God. On Purpose.

Date: _____

You're either going to love yourself or hate yourself. Choose love.
- Queen Latifah

The one thing I'll accomplish to win today is:
_____
_____

The life goal this applies to is:
_____
_____

The skills and talents I will use to do this are:
_____
_____

An empowering thought to help is:
_____
_____

My self-care action for today is:
_____
_____

Other To-Do's:	Today I'm thankful for:

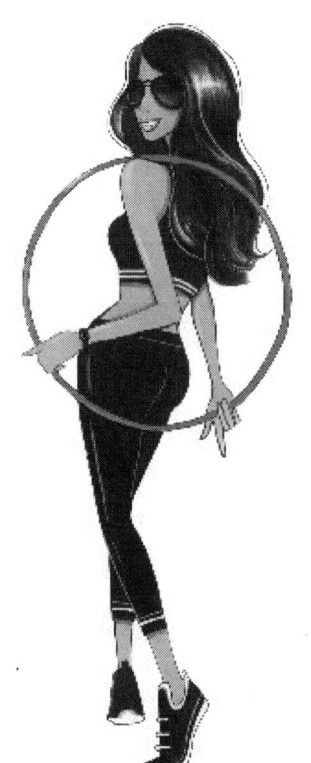

Design Your Happy. With God. On Purpose.

Date: _____

Go in the strength you have...
- Judges 6:14

The one thing I'll accomplish to win today is:
_____
_____

The life goal this applies to is:
_____
_____

The skills and talents I will use to do this are:
_____
_____

An empowering thought to help is:
_____
_____

My self-care action for today is:
_____
_____

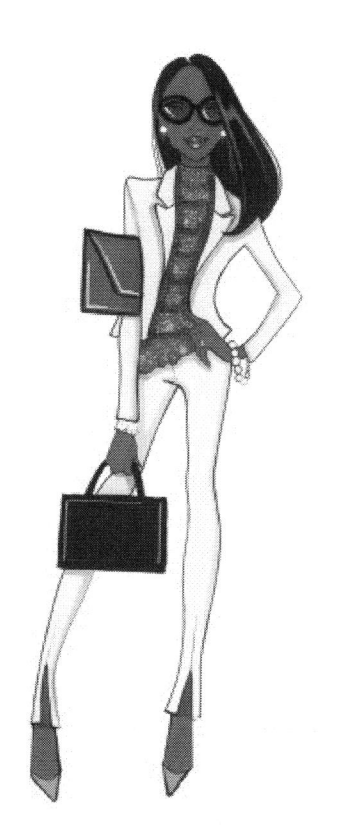

Other To-Do's:	Today I'm thankful for:

Design Your Happy. With God. On Purpose.

Date: _____

Imagination is more important than knowledge.
- Albert Einstein

The one thing I'll accomplish to win today is:
_____
_____

The life goal this applies to is:
_____
_____

The skills and talents I will use to do this are:
_____
_____

An empowering thought to help is:
_____
_____

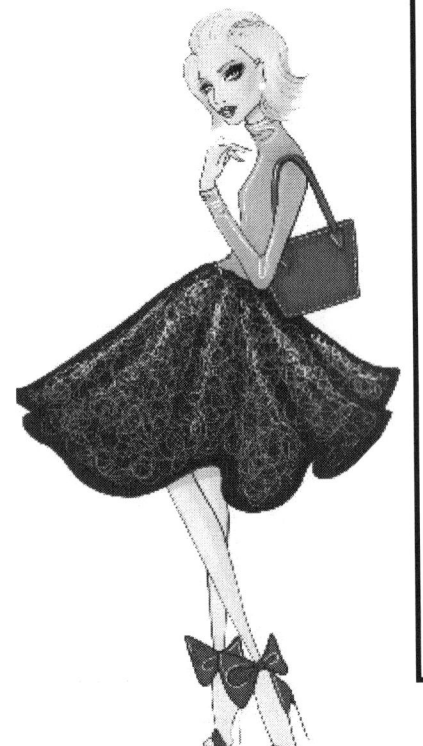

My self-care action for today is:
_____
_____

Other To-Do's:	Today I'm thankful for:

Design Your Happy. With God. On Purpose.

Date: _____

Sometimes you have to break down to break through.
- Betsy Bernard

The one thing I'll accomplish to win today is:
_____
_____

The life goal this applies to is:
_____
_____

The skills and talents I will use to do this are:
_____
_____

An empowering thought to help is:
_____
_____

My self-care action for today is:
_____
_____

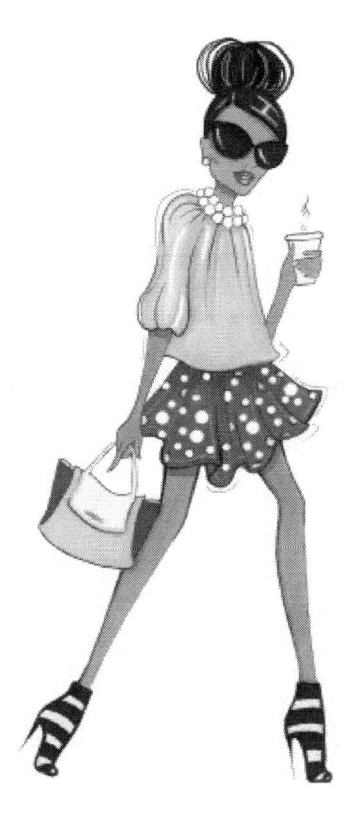

Other To-Do's:	Today I'm thankful for:

Design Your Happy. With God. On Purpose.

Date: _____

Results count, act like you belong and wear the yellow jacket.
- Rebecca Doherty

The one thing I'll accomplish to win today is:
_____
_____

The life goal this applies to is:
_____
_____

The skills and talents I will use to do this are:
_____
_____

An empowering thought to help is:
_____
_____

My self-care action for today is:
_____
_____

Other To-Do's:	Today I'm thankful for:

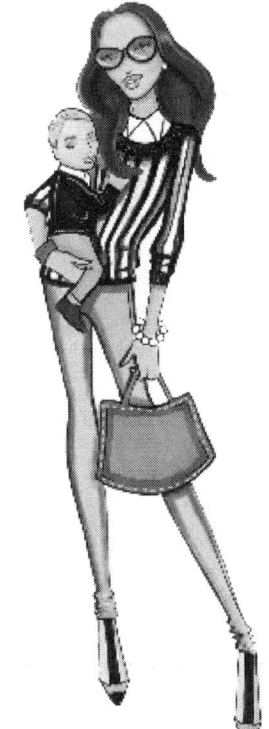

Design Your Happy. With God. On Purpose.

Date: _____

Self-knowledge is the beginning of self-improvement.
- Baltasar Gracian

The one thing I'll accomplish to win today is:
_____
_____

The life goal this applies to is:
_____
_____

The skills and talents I will use to do this are:
_____
_____

An empowering thought to help is:
_____
_____

My self-care action for today is:
_____
_____

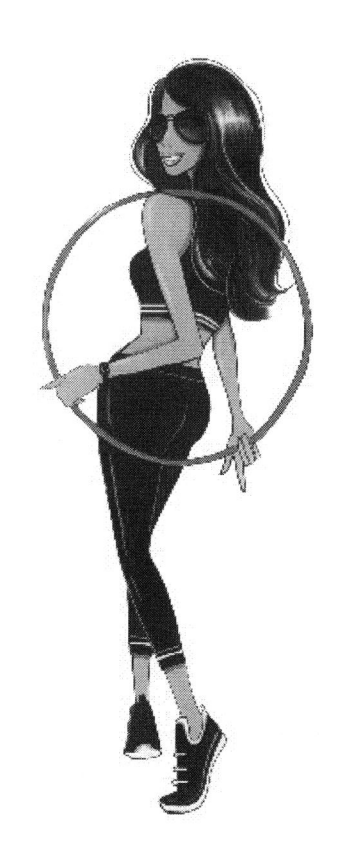

Other To-Do's:	Today I'm thankful for:

Design Your Happy. With God. On Purpose.

Date: _____

Use the influence you have wherever you are.
- Betsy Bernard

The one thing I'll accomplish to win today is:
_____
_____

The life goal this applies to is:
_____
_____

The skills and talents I will use to do this are:
_____
_____

An empowering thought to help is:
_____
_____

My self-care action for today is:
_____
_____

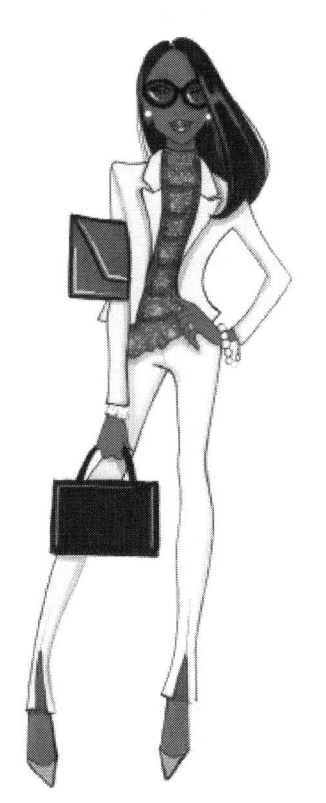

Other To-Do's:	Today I'm thankful for:

Design Your Happy. With God. On Purpose.

Date: _____

The way to a big project is by doing a lot of small ones very well.
- Lynn Marmer

The one thing I'll accomplish to win today is:
_____
_____

The life goal this applies to is:
_____
_____

The skills and talents I will use to do this are:
_____
_____

An empowering thought to help is:
_____
_____

My self-care action for today is:
_____
_____

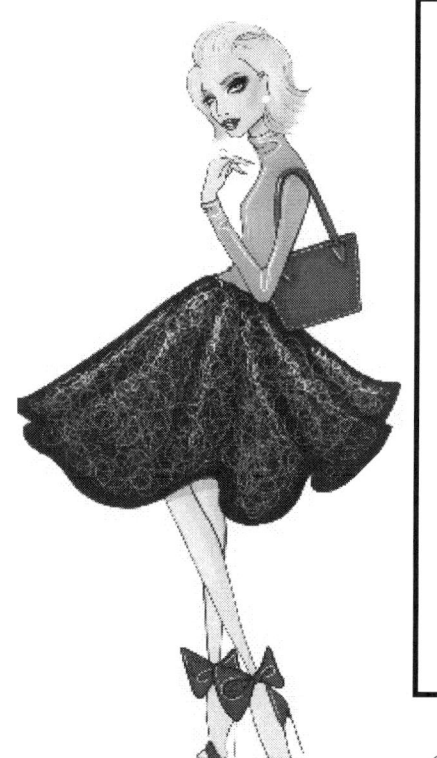

Other To-Do's:	Today I'm thankful for:

Design Your Happy. With God. On Purpose.

Date: _____

Don't be timid about your power. Use it. Risk disapproval.
- Arianna Huffington

The one thing I'll accomplish to win today is:
_____
_____

The life goal this applies to is:
_____
_____

The skills and talents I will use to do this are:
_____
_____

An empowering thought to help is:
_____
_____

My self-care action for today is:
_____
_____

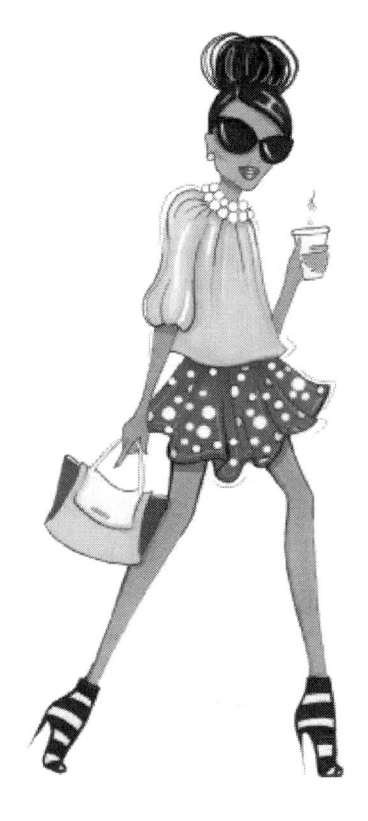

Other To-Do's:	Today I'm thankful for:

Design Your Happy. With God. On Purpose.

Date: _____

It's important to seize wonderful moments as they happen.
- Mary-Ellis Bunim

The one thing I'll accomplish to win today is:
_____
_____

The life goal this applies to is:
_____
_____

The skills and talents I will use to do this are:
_____
_____

An empowering thought to help is:
_____
_____

My self-care action for today is:
_____
_____

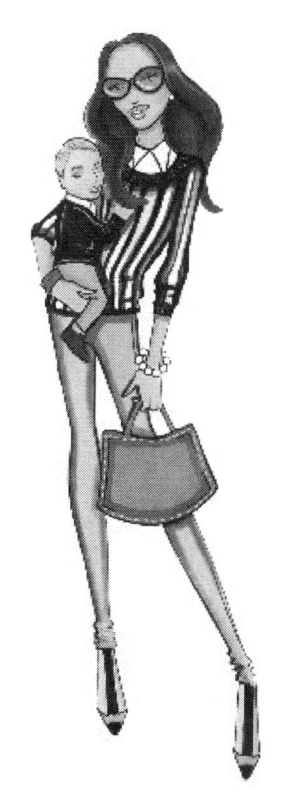

Other To-Do's:	Today I'm thankful for:

Design Your Happy. With God. On Purpose.

Date: _____

I praise you because I am fearfully and wonderfully made.
- Psalm 139:14

The one thing I'll accomplish to win today is:
_____
_____

The life goal this applies to is:
_____
_____

The skills and talents I will use to do this are:
_____
_____

An empowering thought to help is:
_____
_____

My self-care action for today is:
_____
_____

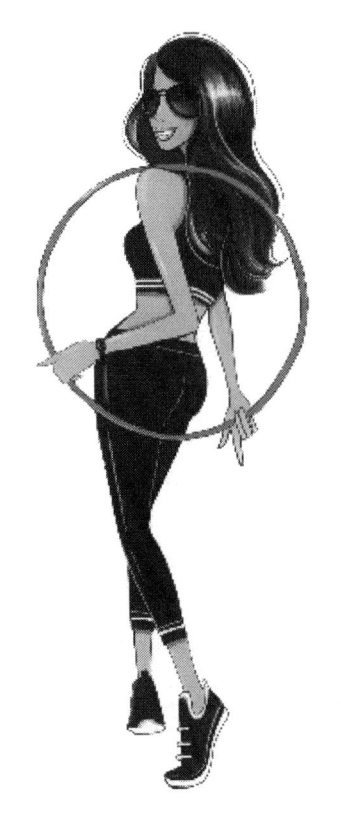

Other To-Do's:	Today I'm thankful for:

Design Your Happy. With God. On Purpose.

Date: _____

The most valuable thing anyone can spend is time.
- Theophrastus

The one thing I'll accomplish to win today is:
_____
_____

The life goal this applies to is:
_____
_____

The skills and talents I will use to do this are:
_____
_____

An empowering thought to help is:
_____
_____

My self-care action for today is:
_____
_____

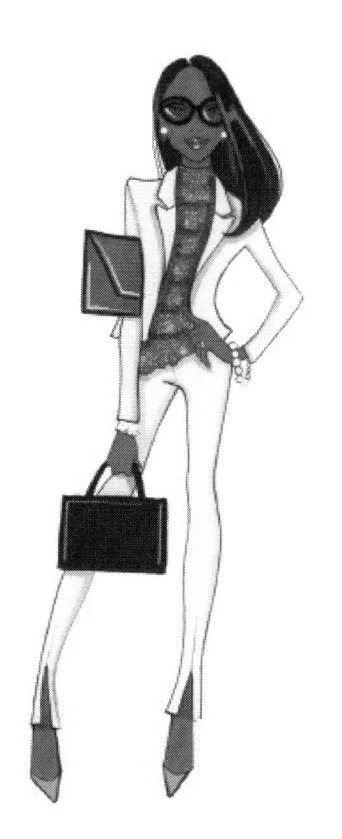

Other To-Do's:	Today I'm thankful for:

Design Your Happy. With God. On Purpose.

Date: _____

Champions are built on a thousand invisible mornings.
- Kirk Cousins

The one thing I'll accomplish to win today is:
_____
_____

The life goal this applies to is:
_____
_____

The skills and talents I will use to do this are:
_____
_____

An empowering thought to help is:
_____
_____

My self-care action for today is:
_____
_____

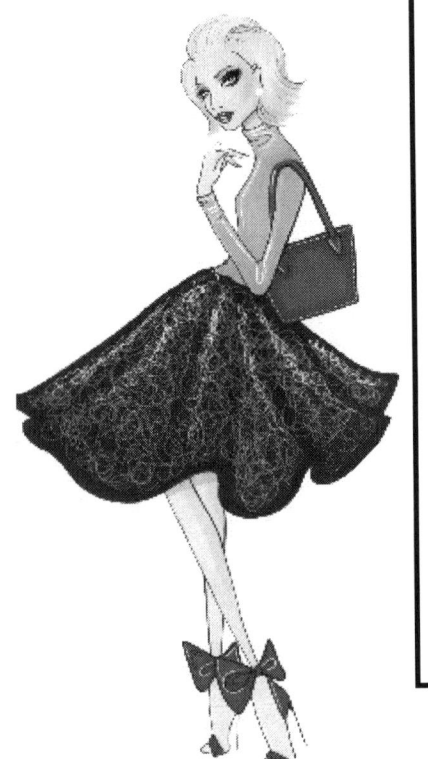

Other To-Do's:	Today I'm thankful for:

Design Your Happy. With God. On Purpose.

Date: _____

Courage is the price life exacts for granting peace
- Amelia Earhart

The one thing I'll accomplish to win today is:
_____
_____

The life goal this applies to is:
_____
_____

The skills and talents I will use to do this are:
_____
_____

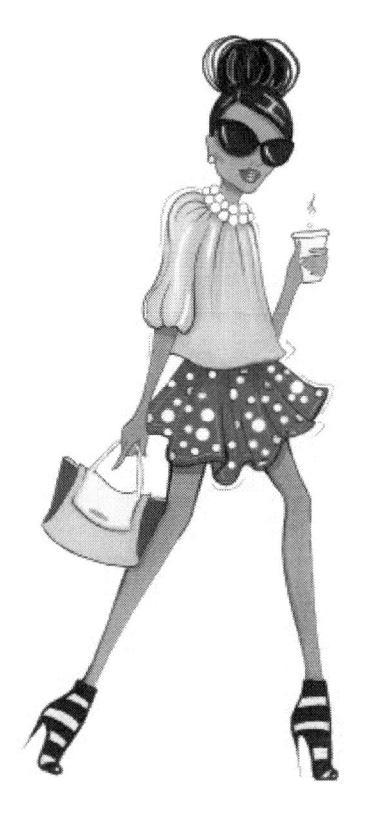

An empowering thought to help is:
_____
_____

My self-care action for today is:
_____
_____

Other To-Do's:	Today I'm thankful for:

Design Your Happy. With God. On Purpose.

Date: _____

Forever is composed of nows.
- Emily Dickinson

The one thing I'll accomplish to win today is:
_____
_____

The life goal this applies to is:
_____
_____

The skills and talents I will use to do this are:
_____
_____

An empowering thought to help is:
_____
_____

My self-care action for today is:
_____
_____

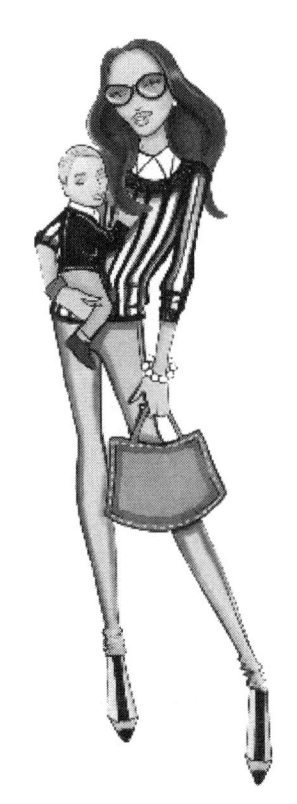

Other To-Do's:	Today I'm thankful for:

Design Your Happy. With God. On Purpose.

Date: _____

Giving up is way harder than trying.
- Kanye

The one thing I'll accomplish to win today is:
_____
_____

The life goal this applies to is:
_____
_____

The skills and talents I will use to do this are:
_____
_____

An empowering thought to help is:
_____
_____

My self-care action for today is:
_____
_____

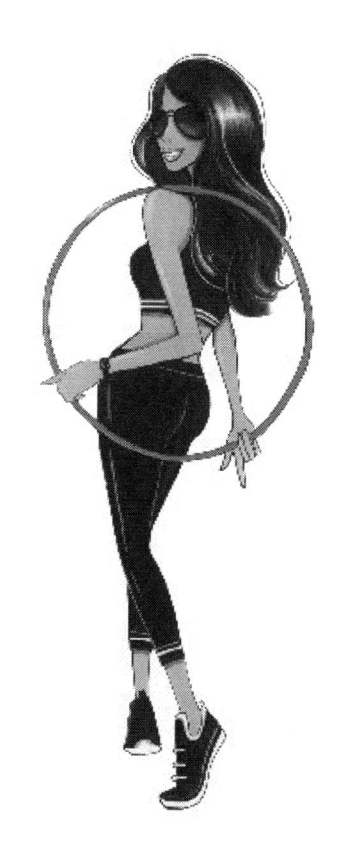

Other To-Do's:	Today I'm thankful for:

Design Your Happy. With God. On Purpose.

Date: _____

The secret of getting ahead is getting started.
- Mark Twain

The one thing I'll accomplish to win today is:
_____
_____

The life goal this applies to is:
_____
_____

The skills and talents I will use to do this are:
_____
_____

An empowering thought to help is:
_____
_____

My self-care action for today is:
_____
_____

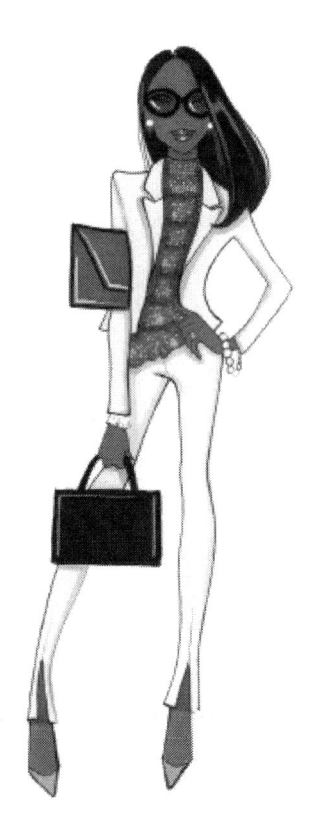

Other To-Do's:	Today I'm thankful for:

Design Your Happy. With God. On Purpose.

Date: _____

We meet no ordinary people in our lives.
- C.S. Lewis

The one thing I'll accomplish to win today is:
_____
_____

The life goal this applies to is:
_____
_____

The skills and talents I will use to do this are:
_____
_____

An empowering thought to help is:
_____
_____

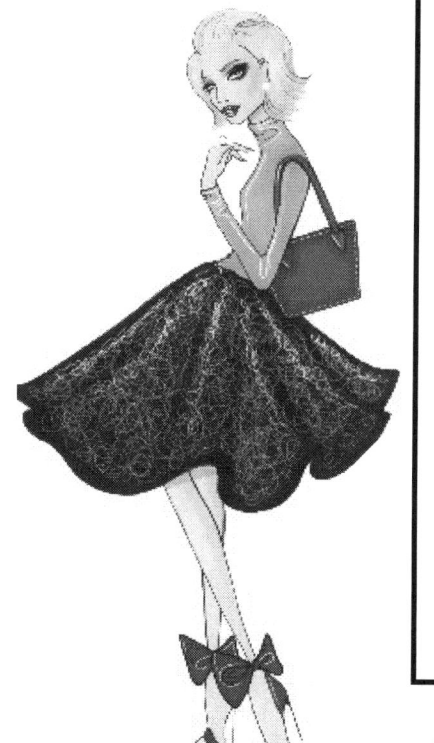

My self-care action for today is:
_____
_____

Other To-Do's:	Today I'm thankful for:

Design Your Happy. With God. On Purpose.

Date: _____

No effort we make to attain something beautiful is ever lost.
- Helen Keller

The one thing I'll accomplish to win today is:
_____
_____

The life goal this applies to is:
_____
_____

The skills and talents I will use to do this are:
_____
_____

An empowering thought to help is:
_____
_____

My self-care action for today is:
_____
_____

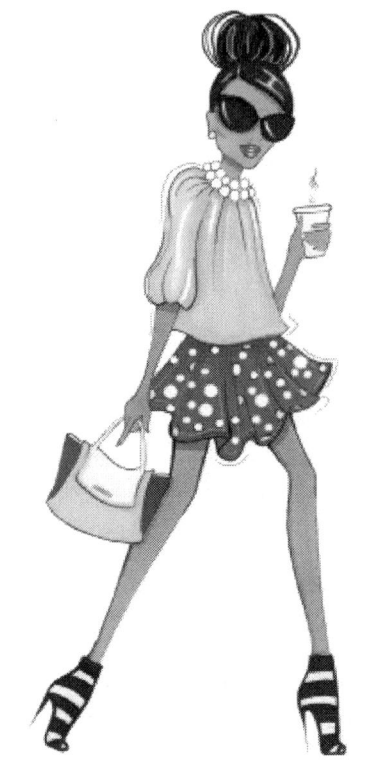

Other To-Do's:	Today I'm thankful for:

Design Your Happy. With God. On Purpose.

Date: _____

If you get, give. If you learn, teach.
- Maya Angelou

The one thing I'll accomplish to win today is:
_____
_____

The life goal this applies to is:
_____
_____

The skills and talents I will use to do this are:
_____
_____

An empowering thought to help is:
_____
_____

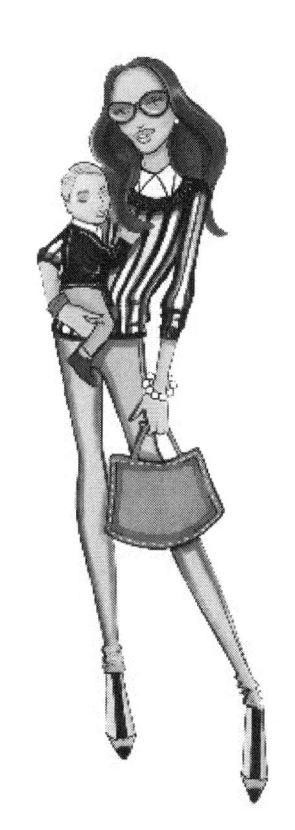

My self-care action for today is:
_____
_____

Other To-Do's:	Today I'm thankful for:

Design Your Happy. With God. On Purpose.

Date: _____

Done is better than perfect.
- Sheryl Sandberg

The one thing I'll accomplish to win today is:
_____
_____

The life goal this applies to is:
_____
_____

The skills and talents I will use to do this are:
_____
_____

An empowering thought to help is:
_____
_____

My self-care action for today is:
_____
_____

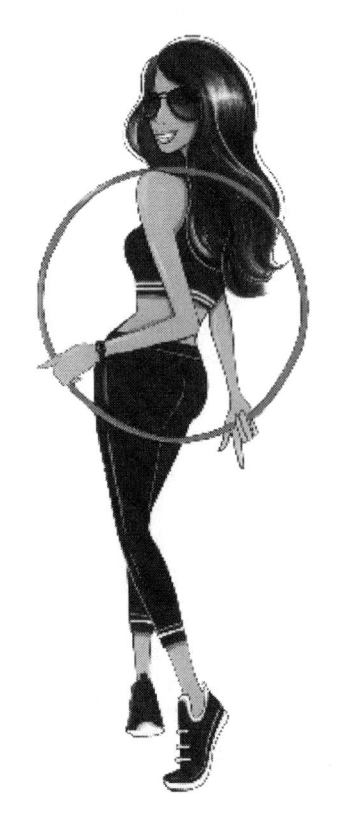

Other To-Do's:	Today I'm thankful for:

Design Your Happy. With God. On Purpose.

Date: _____

Every new beginning comes from some other beginning's end.
- Seneca

The one thing I'll accomplish to win today is:
_____
_____

The life goal this applies to is:
_____
_____

The skills and talents I will use to do this are:
_____
_____

An empowering thought to help is:
_____
_____

My self-care action for today is:
_____
_____

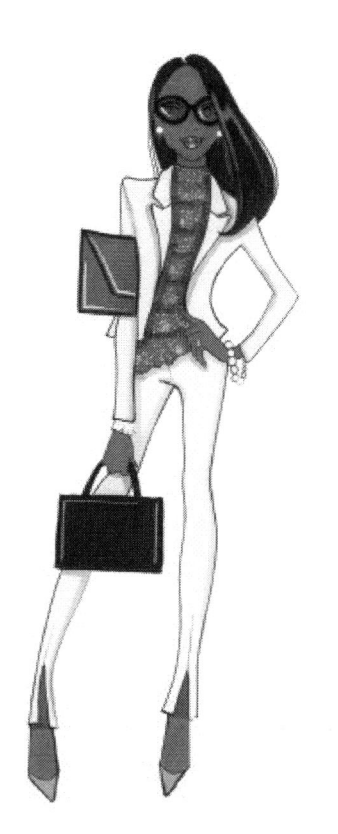

Other To-Do's:	Today I'm thankful for:

Design Your Happy. With God. On Purpose.

Date: _____

Better three hours too soon than a minute too late.
- William Shakespeare

The one thing I'll accomplish to win today is:
_____
_____

The life goal this applies to is:
_____
_____

The skills and talents I will use to do this are:
_____
_____

An empowering thought to help is:
_____
_____

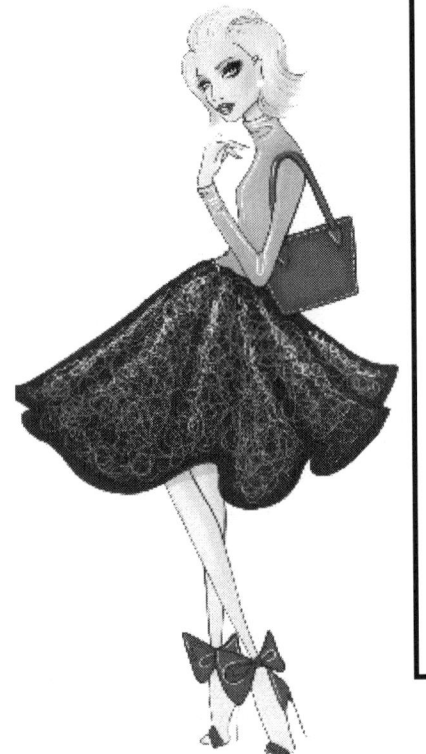

My self-care action for today is:
_____
_____

Other To-Do's:	Today I'm thankful for:

Design Your Happy. With God. On Purpose.

Date: _____

The only recognizable feature of hope is action.
- Grace Paley

The one thing I'll accomplish to win today is:
_____
_____

The life goal this applies to is:
_____
_____

The skills and talents I will use to do this are:
_____
_____

An empowering thought to help is:
_____
_____

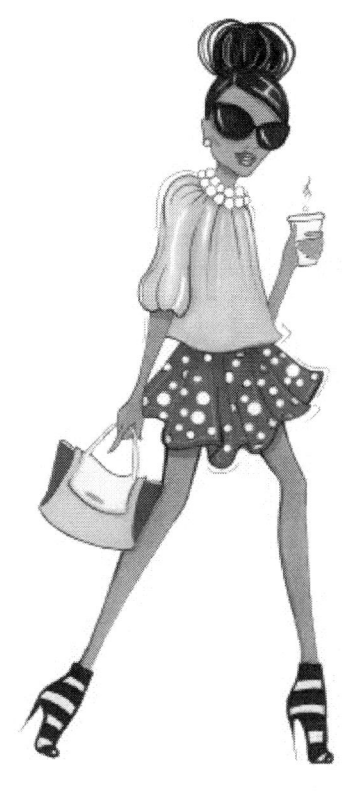

My self-care action for today is:
_____
_____

Other To-Do's:	Today I'm thankful for:

Design Your Happy. With God. On Purpose.

Date: _____

But those who hope in the Lord will renew their strength.
- Isaiah 40:31

The one thing I'll accomplish to win today is:

_____
_____

The life goal this applies to is:

_____
_____

The skills and talents I will use to do this are:

_____
_____

An empowering thought to help is:

_____
_____

My self-care action for today is:

_____
_____

Other To-Do's:	Today I'm thankful for:

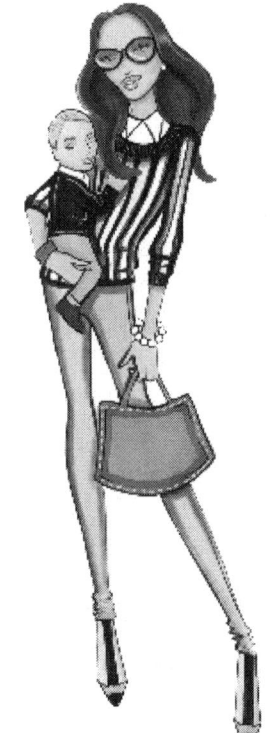

Design Your Happy. With God. On Purpose.

Date: _____

If you have hope, you can have courage.
- Katherine Switzer

The one thing I'll accomplish to win today is:
_____
_____

The life goal this applies to is:
_____
_____

The skills and talents I will use to do this are:
_____
_____

An empowering thought to help is:
_____
_____

My self-care action for today is:
_____
_____

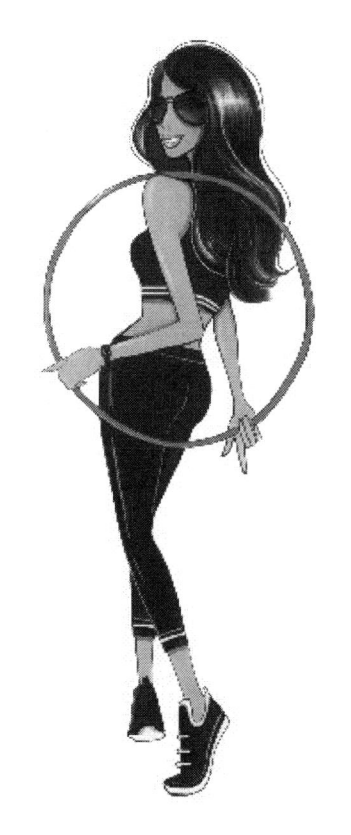

Other To-Do's:	Today I'm thankful for:

Design Your Happy. With God. On Purpose.

Date: _____

I had to get over my fear of not being liked.
- Dr. Christiane Northrup

The one thing I'll accomplish to win today is:
_____
_____

The life goal this applies to is:
_____
_____

The skills and talents I will use to do this are:
_____
_____

An empowering thought to help is:
_____
_____

My self-care action for today is:
_____
_____

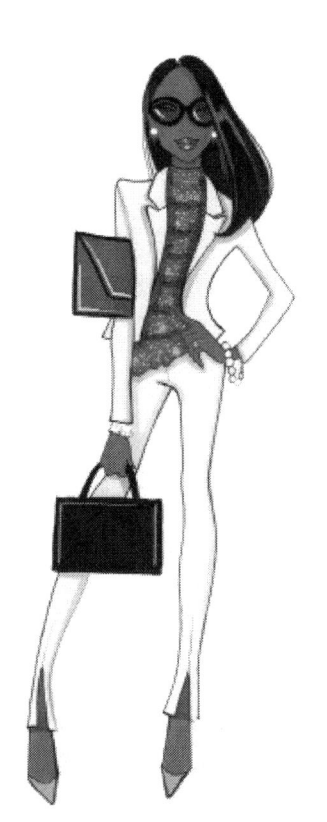

Other To-Do's:	Today I'm thankful for:

Design Your Happy. With God. On Purpose.

Date: _____

The day you see the truth and cease to speak is the day you die.
- Jocelyn Elders

The one thing I'll accomplish to win today is:
_____
_____

The life goal this applies to is:
_____
_____

The skills and talents I will use to do this are:
_____
_____

An empowering thought to help is:
_____
_____

My self-care action for today is:
_____
_____

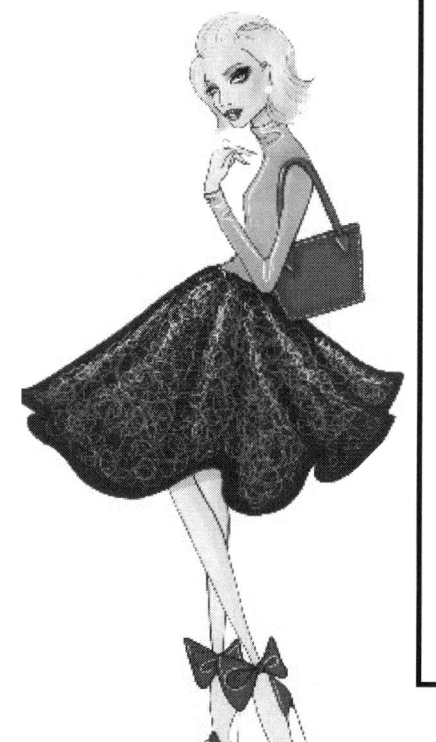

Other To-Do's:	Today I'm thankful for:

Design Your Happy. With God. On Purpose.

Date: _____

Ask what you don't know.
- Meg Whitman

The one thing I'll accomplish to win today is:
_____
_____

The life goal this applies to is:
_____
_____

The skills and talents I will use to do this are:
_____
_____

An empowering thought to help is:
_____
_____

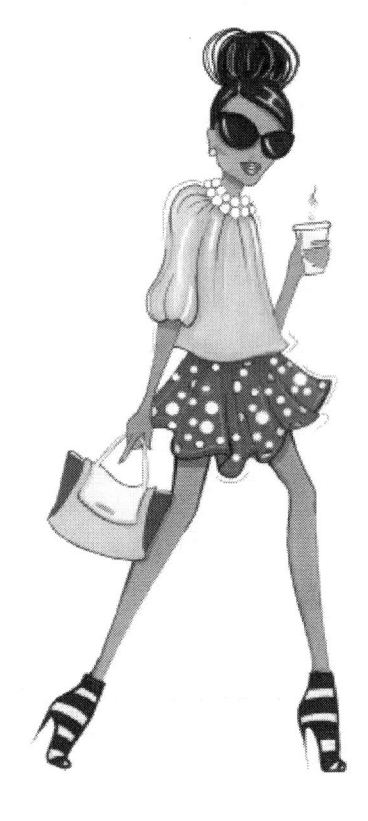

My self-care action for today is:
_____
_____

Other To-Do's:	Today I'm thankful for:

Design Your Happy. With God. On Purpose.

Date: _____

No pressure, no diamonds.
- Thomas Carlyle

The one thing I'll accomplish to win today is:
_____
_____

The life goal this applies to is:
_____
_____

The skills and talents I will use to do this are:
_____
_____

An empowering thought to help is:
_____
_____

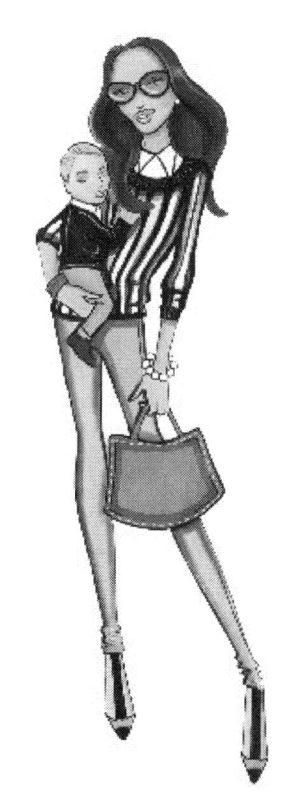

My self-care action for today is:
_____
_____

Other To-Do's:	Today I'm thankful for:

Design Your Happy. With God. On Purpose.

Date: _____

Without fear there is no courage.
- Chantelle Anderson

The one thing I'll accomplish to win today is:
_____
_____

The life goal this applies to is:
_____
_____

The skills and talents I will use to do this are:
_____
_____

An empowering thought to help is:
_____
_____

My self-care action for today is:
_____
_____

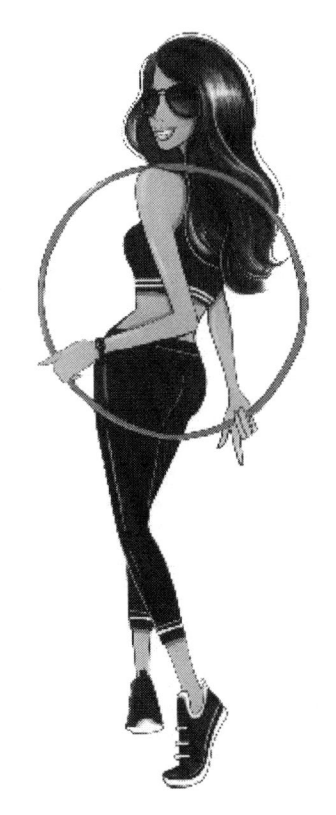

Other To-Do's:	Today I'm thankful for:

Design Your Happy. With God. On Purpose.

Date: _____

Everything has beauty but not everyone sees it.
- Confucius

The one thing I'll accomplish to win today is:
_____
_____

The life goal this applies to is:
_____
_____

The skills and talents I will use to do this are:
_____
_____

An empowering thought to help is:
_____
_____

My self-care action for today is:
_____
_____

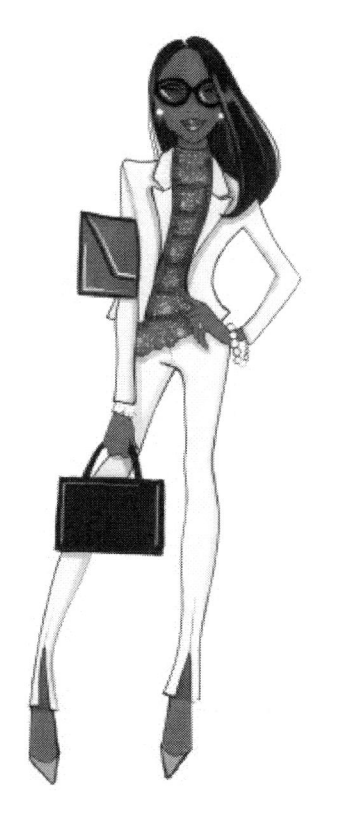

Other To-Do's:	Today I'm thankful for:

Design Your Happy. With God. On Purpose.

Date: _____

Networking is working.
- Denise Morrison

The one thing I'll accomplish to win today is:
_____
_____

The life goal this applies to is:
_____
_____

The skills and talents I will use to do this are:
_____
_____

An empowering thought to help is:
_____
_____

My self-care action for today is:
_____
_____

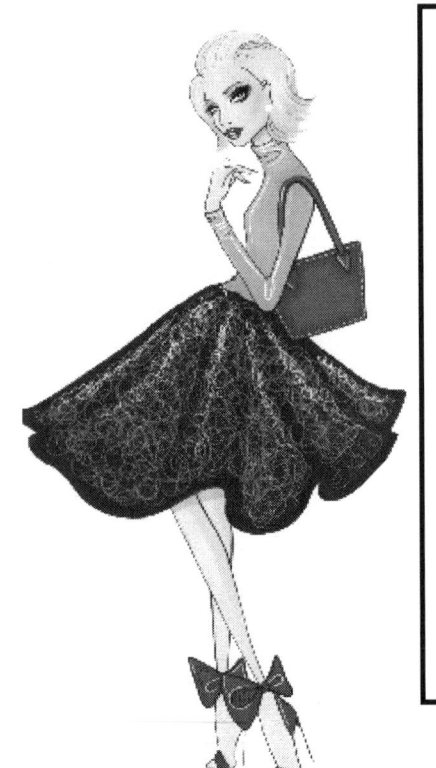

Other To-Do's:	Today I'm thankful for:

Design Your Happy. With God. On Purpose.

Date: _____

Lost time is never found again.
- Benjamin Franklin

The one thing I'll accomplish to win today is:
_____
_____

The life goal this applies to is:
_____
_____

The skills and talents I will use to do this are:
_____
_____

An empowering thought to help is:
_____
_____

My self-care action for today is:
_____
_____

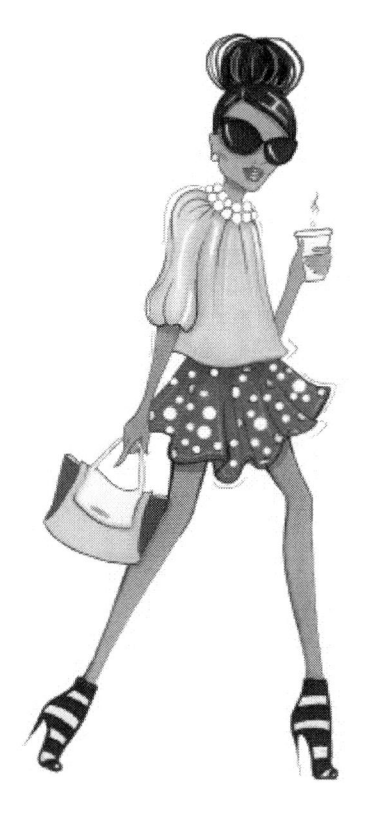

Other To-Do's:	Today I'm thankful for:

Design Your Happy. With God. On Purpose.

Date: _____

Cast all your anxiety on Him because He cares for you.
- 1 Peter 5:7

The one thing I'll accomplish to win today is:
_____
_____

The life goal this applies to is:
_____
_____

The skills and talents I will use to do this are:
_____
_____

An empowering thought to help is:
_____
_____

My self-care action for today is:
_____
_____

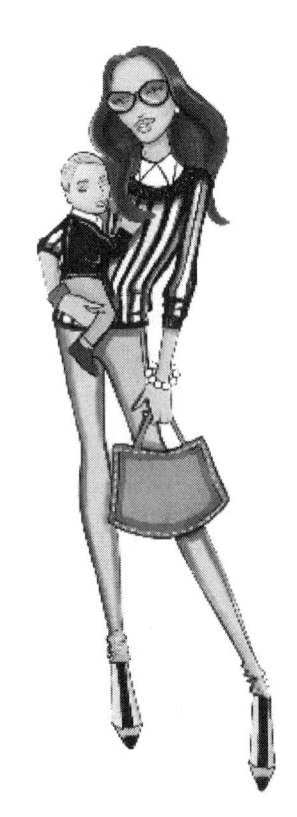

Other To-Do's:	Today I'm thankful for:

Design Your Happy. With God. On Purpose.

Date: _____

Be not afraid of growing slowly. Be afraid of standing still.
- Chinese Proverb

The one thing I'll accomplish to win today is:
_____
_____

The life goal this applies to is:
_____
_____

The skills and talents I will use to do this are:
_____
_____

An empowering thought to help is:
_____
_____

My self-care action for today is:
_____
_____

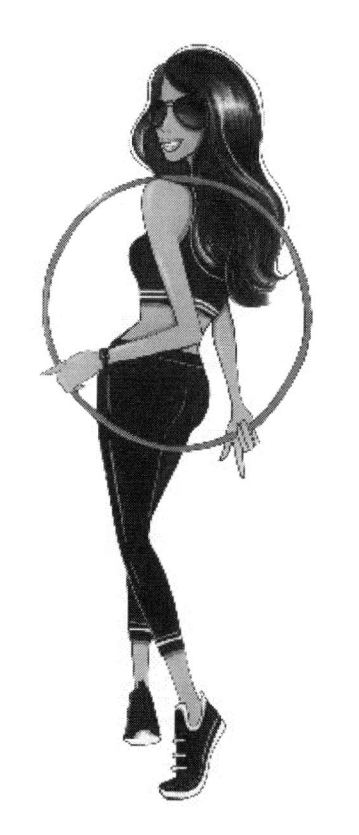

Other To-Do's:	Today I'm thankful for:

Design Your Happy. With God. On Purpose.

Date: _____

Honesty prospers in every condition of life.
- Friedrich Schiller

The one thing I'll accomplish to win today is:

_____
_____

The life goal this applies to is:

_____
_____

The skills and talents I will use to do this are:

_____
_____

An empowering thought to help is:

_____
_____

My self-care action for today is:

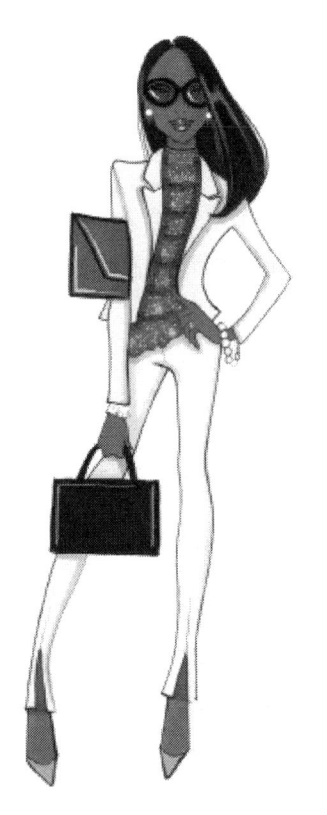

_____
_____

Other To-Do's:	Today I'm thankful for:

Design Your Happy. With God. On Purpose.

Date: _____

Trust your personality.
- Kristin Smith

The one thing I'll accomplish to win today is:
_____
_____

The life goal this applies to is:
_____
_____

The skills and talents I will use to do this are:
_____
_____

An empowering thought to help is:
_____
_____

My self-care action for today is:
_____
_____

Other To-Do's:	Today I'm thankful for:

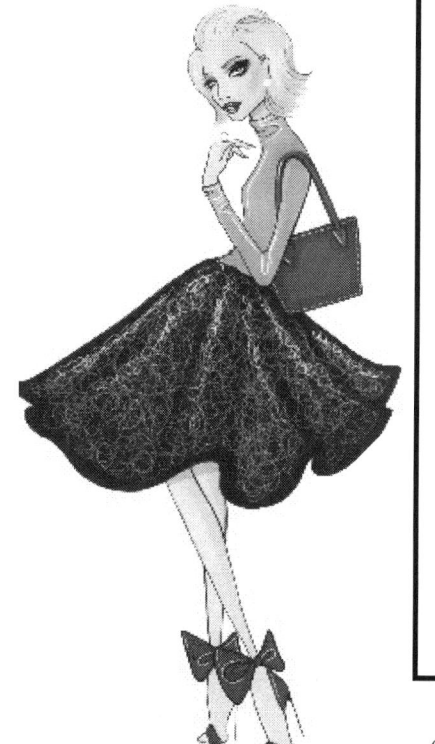

Design Your Happy. With God. On Purpose.

Date: _____

Dream no small dreams, for they have no power to move hearts.
- Von Gothe

The one thing I'll accomplish to win today is:
_____
_____

The life goal this applies to is:
_____
_____

The skills and talents I will use to do this are:
_____
_____

An empowering thought to help is:
_____
_____

My self-care action for today is:
_____
_____

Other To-Do's:	Today I'm thankful for:

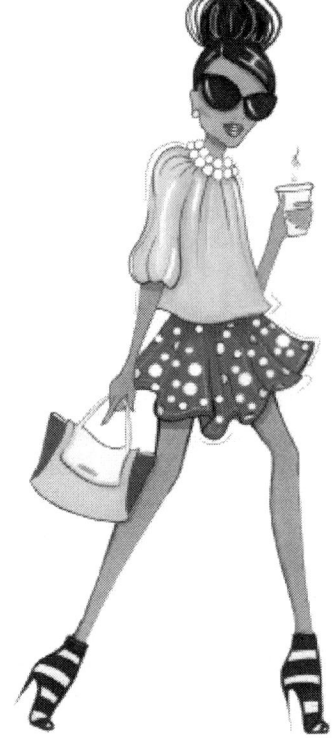

Design Your Happy. With God. On Purpose.

Date: _____

If it is worth doing, it is worth doing right.
- Michelle Gloeckler

The one thing I'll accomplish to win today is:
_____
_____

The life goal this applies to is:
_____
_____

The skills and talents I will use to do this are:
_____
_____

An empowering thought to help is:
_____
_____

My self-care action for today is:
_____
_____

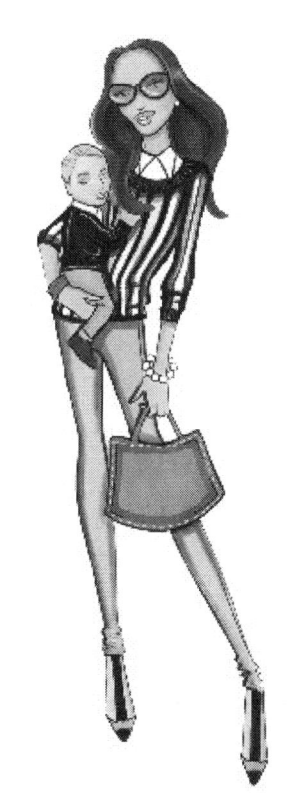

Other To-Do's:	Today I'm thankful for:

Design Your Happy. With God. On Purpose.

Date: _____

You have to know, every day, that you are proud of what you did.
- Joan Toth

The one thing I'll accomplish to win today is:
_____
_____

The life goal this applies to is:
_____
_____

The skills and talents I will use to do this are:
_____
_____

An empowering thought to help is:
_____
_____

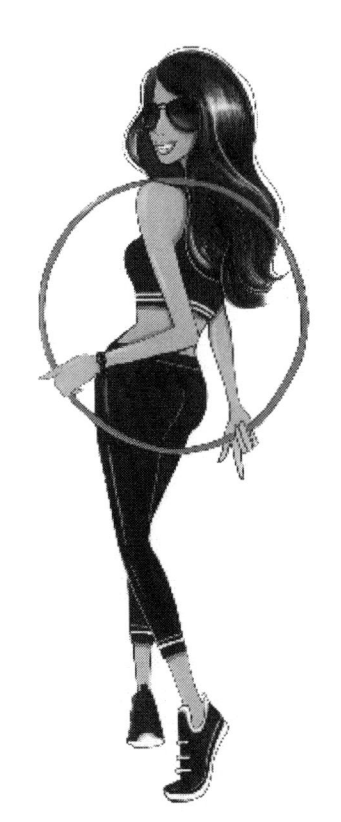

My self-care action for today is:
_____
_____

Other To-Do's:	Today I'm thankful for:

Design Your Happy. With God. On Purpose.

Date: _____

Life shrinks or expands in proportion to one's courage.
- Anais Nin

The one thing I'll accomplish to win today is:
_____
_____

The life goal this applies to is:
_____
_____

The skills and talents I will use to do this are:
_____
_____

An empowering thought to help is:
_____
_____

My self-care action for today is:
_____
_____

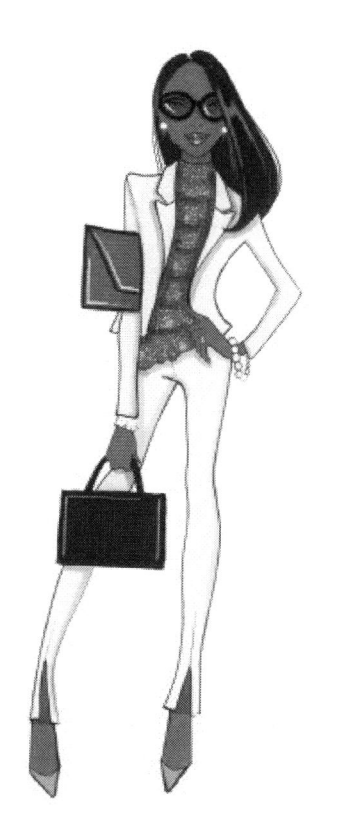

Other To-Do's:	Today I'm thankful for:

Design Your Happy. With God. On Purpose.

Date: _____

The light was in the darkness...the darkness did not overcome it.
- John 1:5

The one thing I'll accomplish to win today is:
_____
_____

The life goal this applies to is:
_____
_____

The skills and talents I will use to do this are:
_____
_____

An empowering thought to help is:
_____
_____

My self-care action for today is:
_____
_____

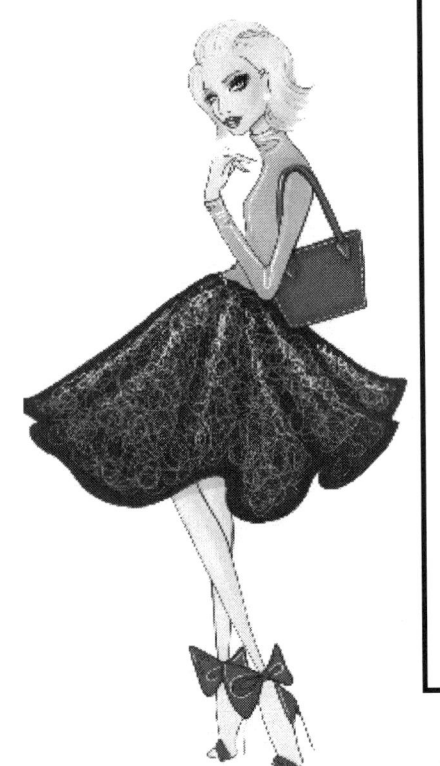

Other To-Do's:	Today I'm thankful for:

Design Your Happy. With God. On Purpose.

Notes from the Journey

Design Your Happy. With God. On Purpose.

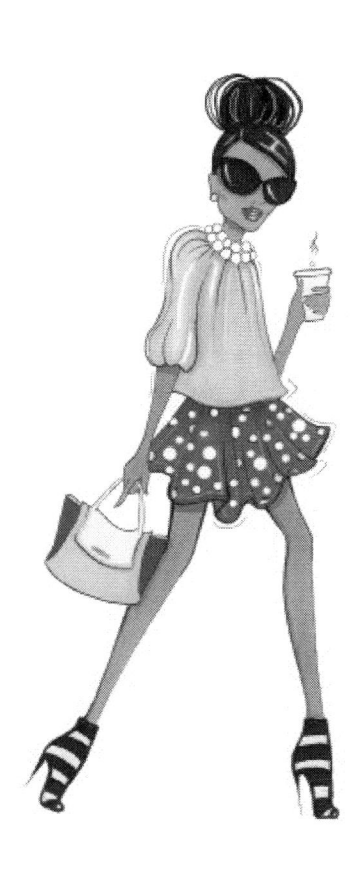

Design Your Happy. With God. On Purpose.

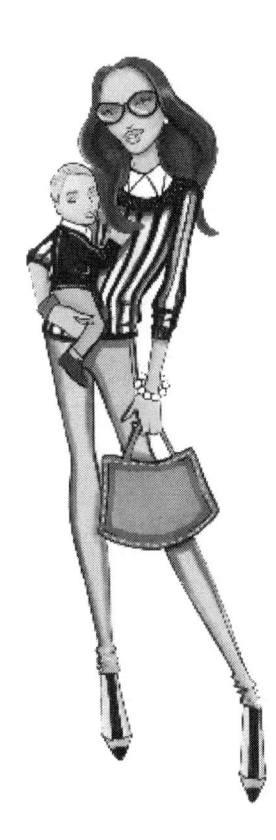

Design Your Happy. With God. On Purpose.

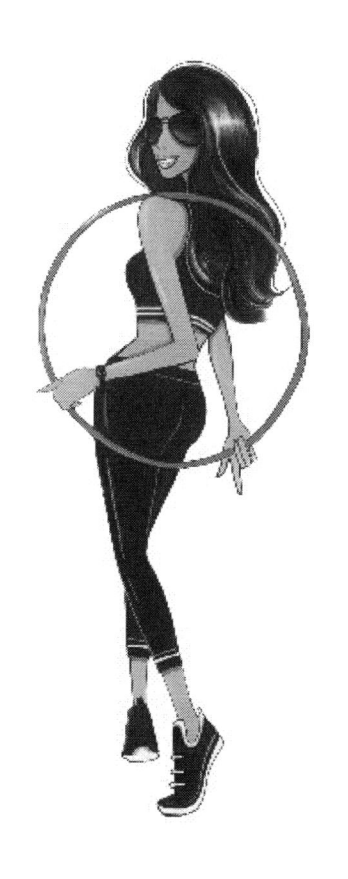

Design Your Happy. With God. On Purpose.

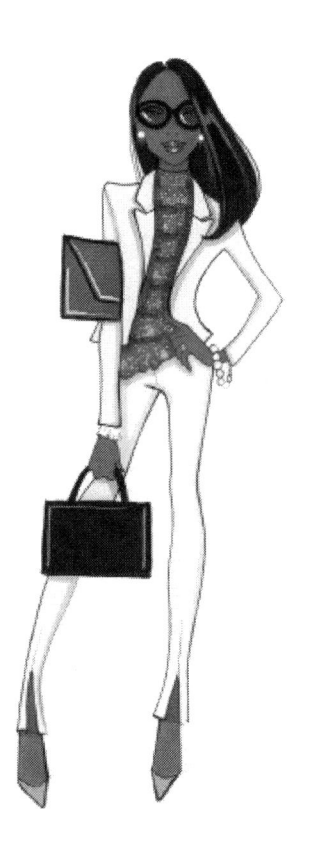

Design Your Happy. With God. On Purpose.

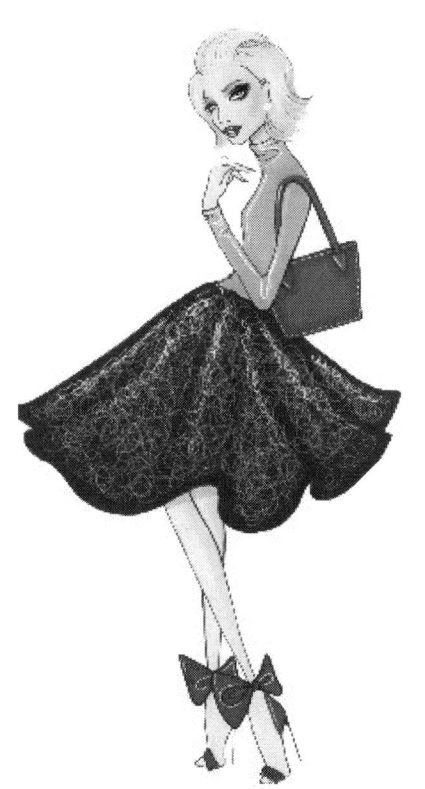

Design Your Happy. With God. On Purpose.

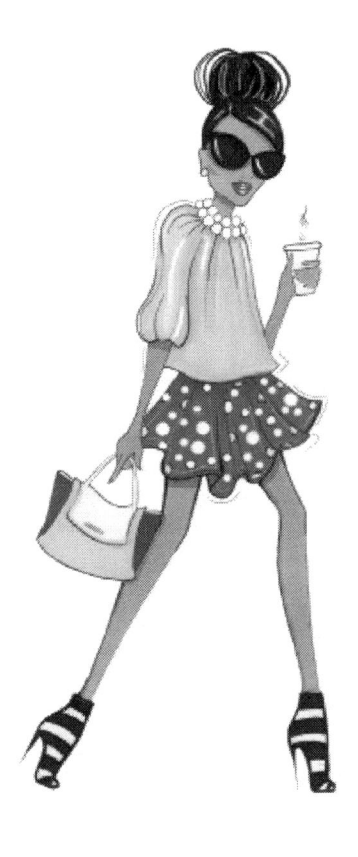

Design Your Happy. With God. On Purpose.

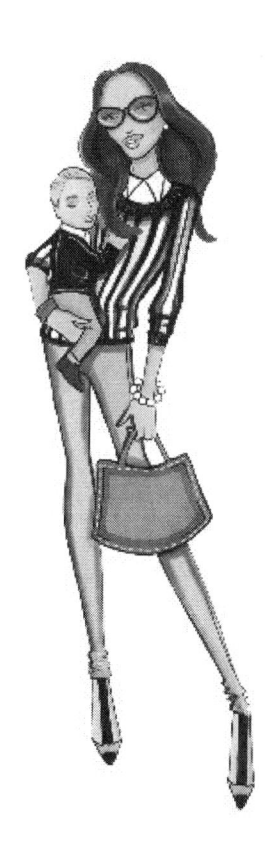

Design Your Happy. With God. On Purpose.

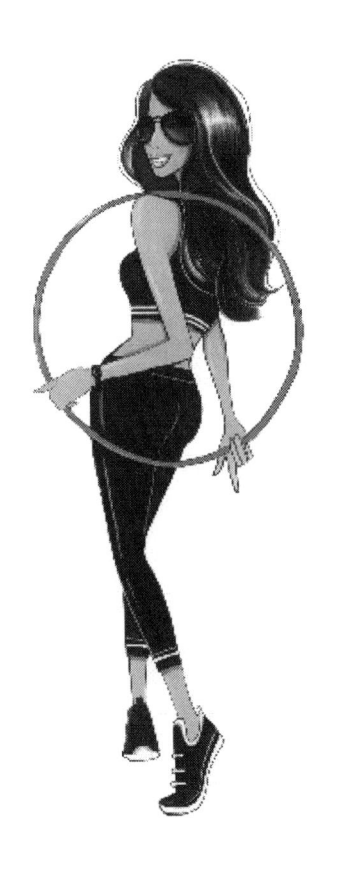

Design Your Happy. With God. On Purpose.

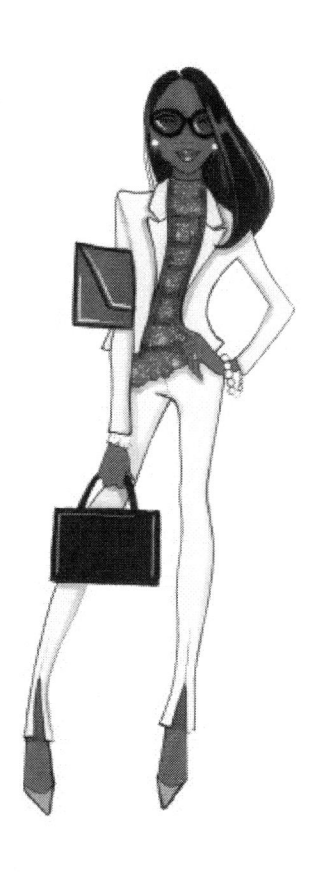

Design Your Happy. With God. On Purpose.

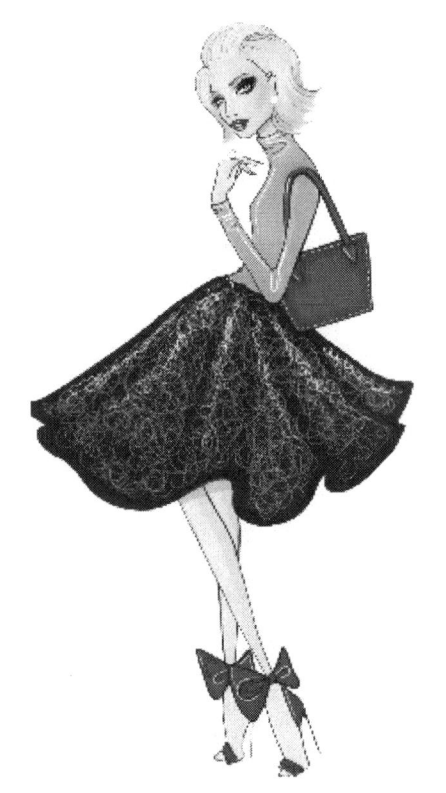

Design Your Happy. With God. On Purpose.

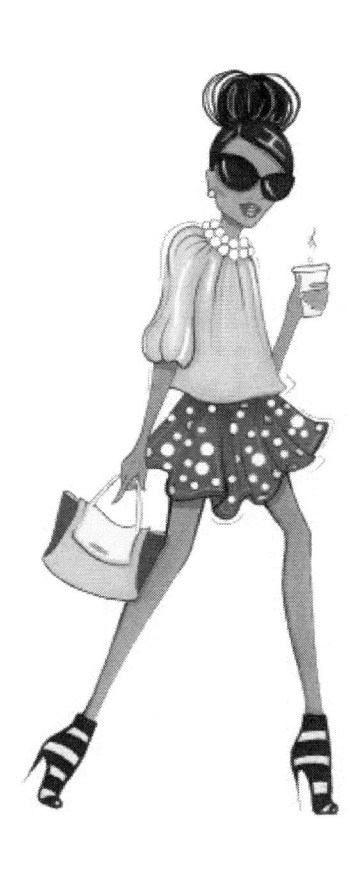

Design Your Happy. With God. On Purpose.

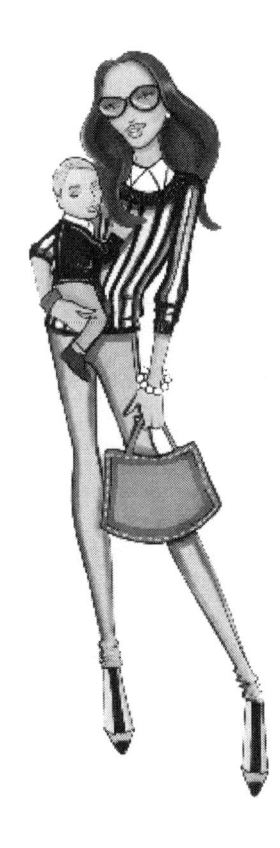

Design Your Happy. With God. On Purpose.

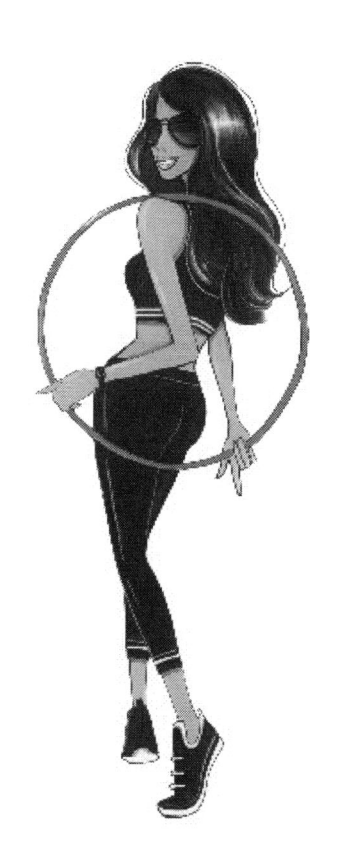

Design Your Happy. With God. On Purpose.

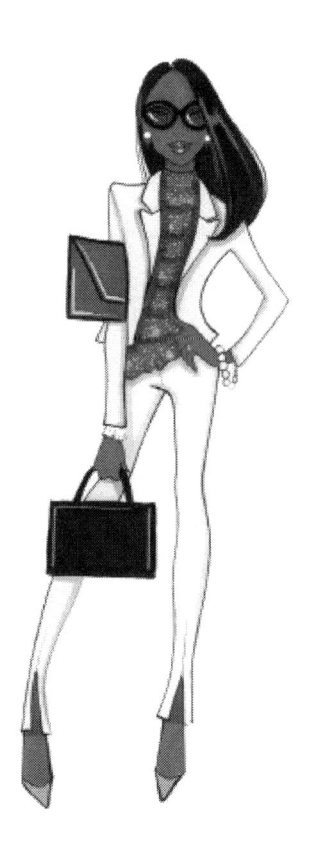

Design Your Happy. With God. On Purpose.

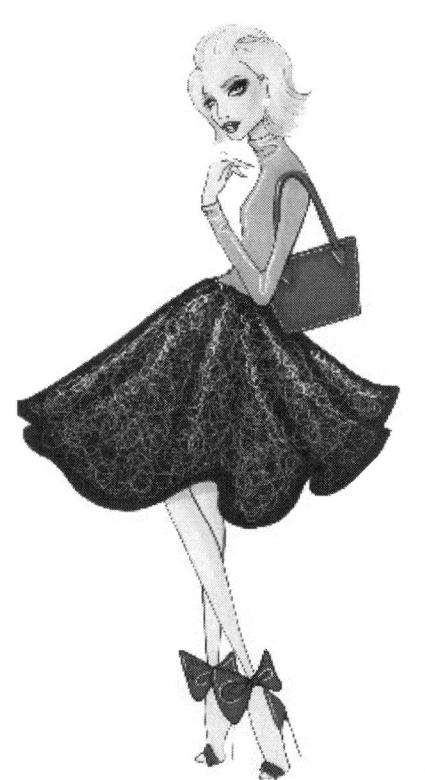

Design Your Happy. With God. On Purpose.

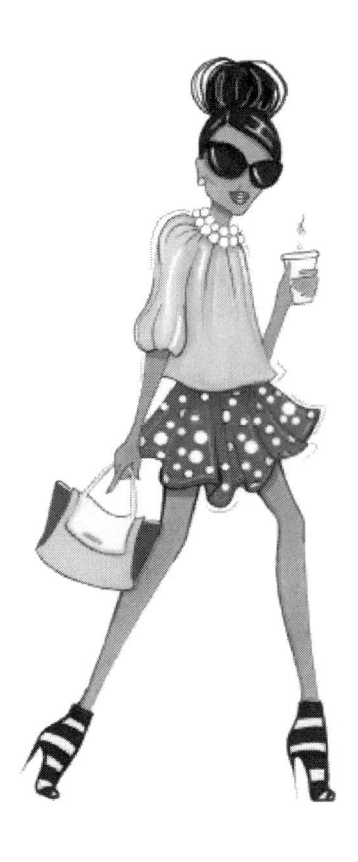

Design Your Happy. With God. On Purpose.

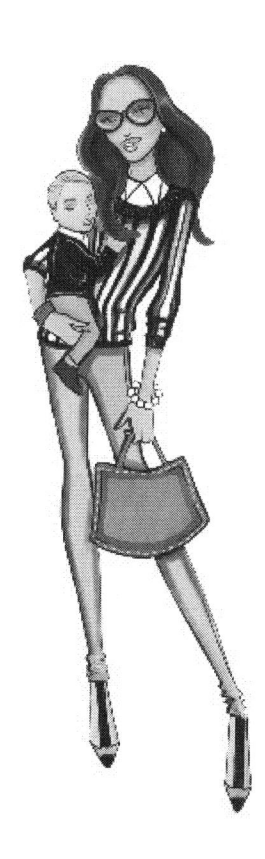

Design Your Happy. With God. On Purpose.

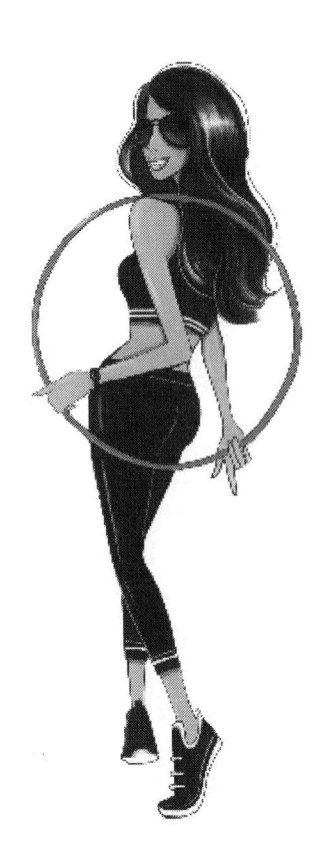

Design Your Happy. With God. On Purpose.

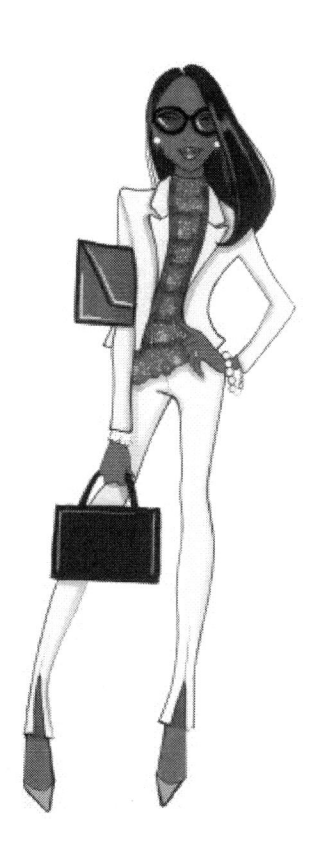

Design Your Happy. With God. On Purpose.

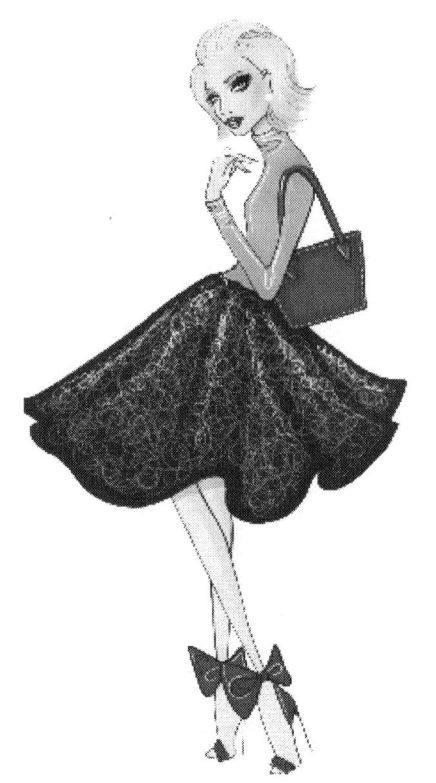

Made in the USA
Columbia, SC
22 December 2019